The Naughty List

The Naughty List welcomes you and hope you will enjoy the following naughty calendar filled with naughty coupons.

Also You will find that on each day there is a different sex position.

The challenge is to climax in THAT position.

(Although during the act you can choose whichever positions you like since all roads lead to rome)

© Copyright 2022 The Naughty List - All rights reserved.

This document is geared towards providing exact and reliable information in regards to the topic and issue covered. The publication is sold with the idea that the publisher is not required to render accounting, officially permitted, or otherwise, qualified services. If advice is necessary, legal or professional, a practiced individual in the profession should be ordered.

- From a Declaration of Principles which was accepted and approved equally by a Committee of the American Bar Association and a Committee of Publishers and Associations.

In no way is it legal to reproduce, duplicate, or transmit any part of this document in either electronic means or in printed format. Recording of this publication is strictly prohibited and any storage of this document is not allowed unless with written permission from the publisher. All rights reserved.

The information provided herein is stated to be truthful and consistent, in that any liability, in terms of inattention or otherwise, by any usage or abuse of any policies, processes, or directions contained within is the solitary and utter responsibility of the recipient reader. Under no circumstances will any legal responsibility or blame be held against the publisher for any reparation, damages, or monetary loss due to the information herein, either directly or indirectly.

Respective authors own all copyrights not held by the publisher.
The information herein is offered for informational purposes solely, and is universal as so. The presentation of the information is without contract or any type of guarantee assurance.

The trademarks that are used are without any consent, and the publication of the trademark is without permission or backing by the trademark owner. All trademarks and brands within this book are for clarifying purposes only and are the owned by the owners themselves, not affiliated with this document.

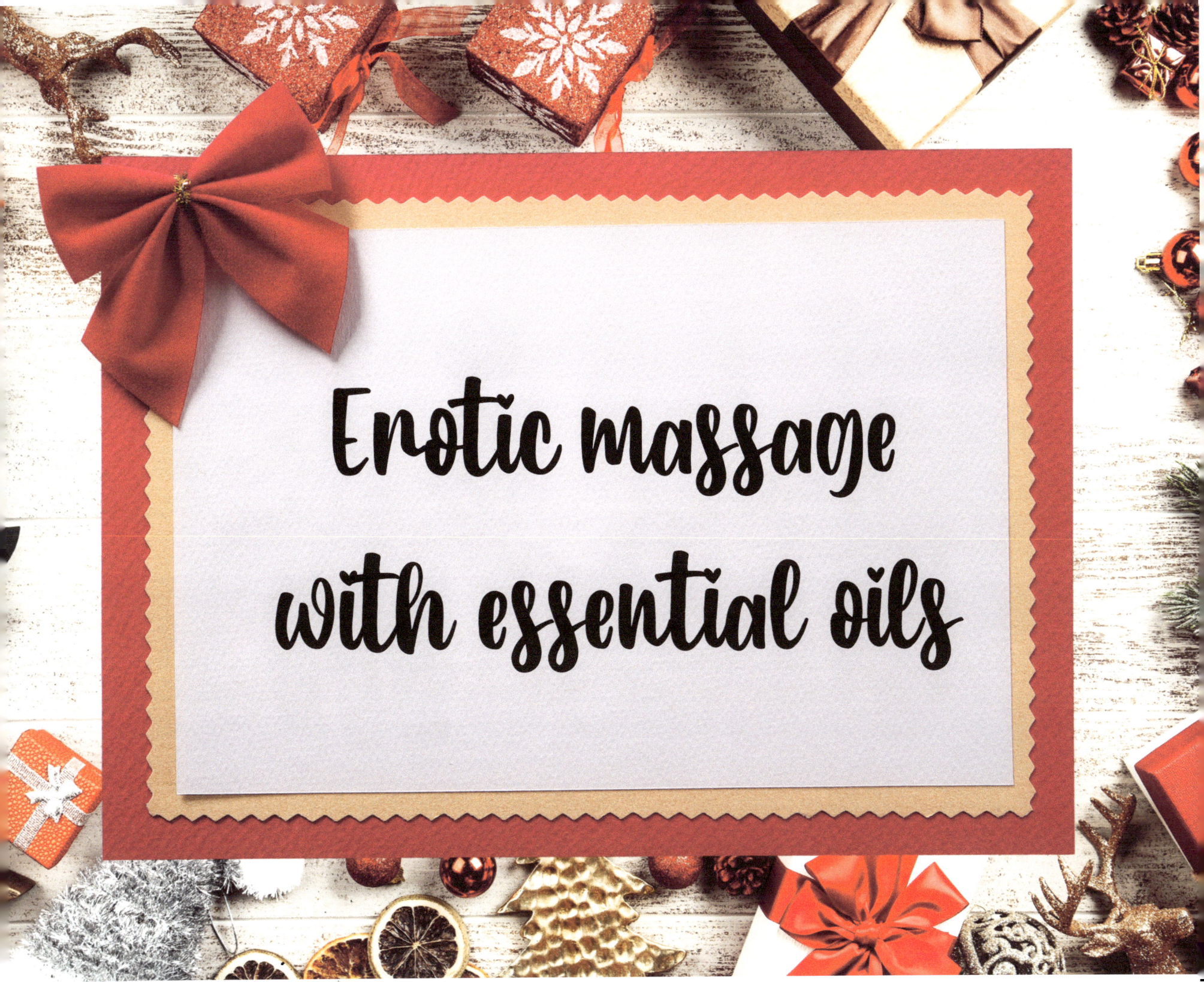

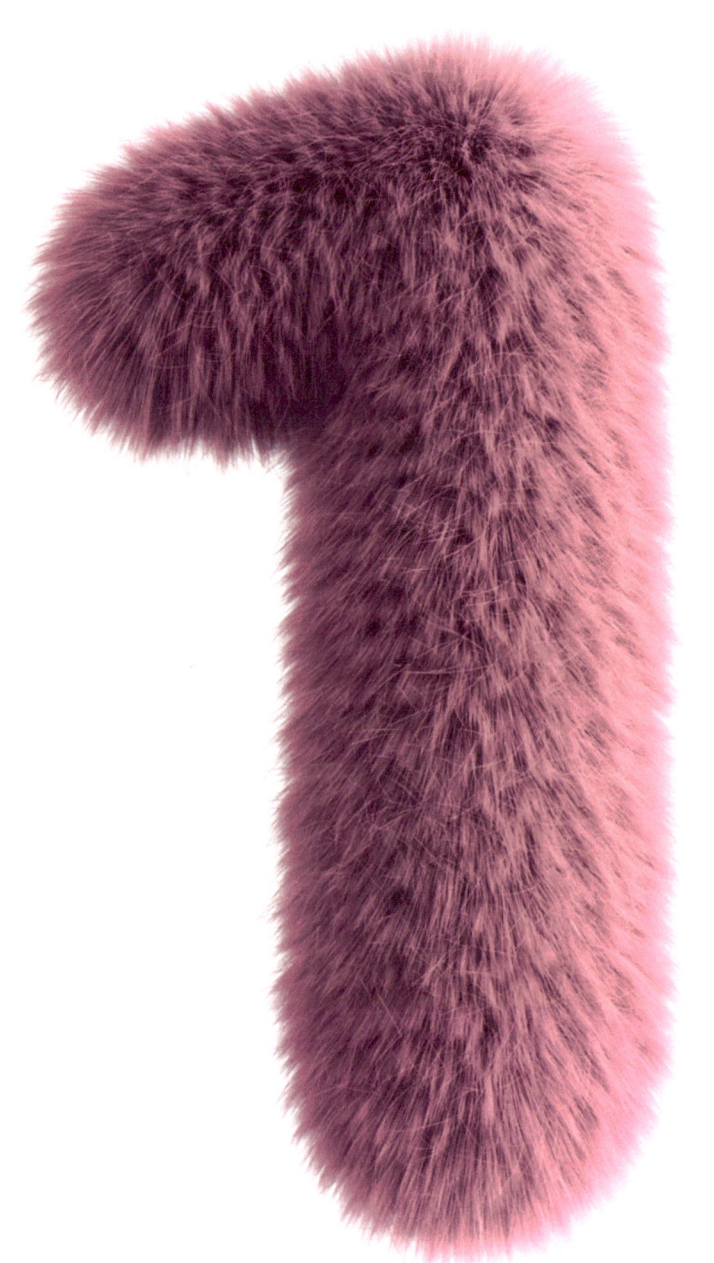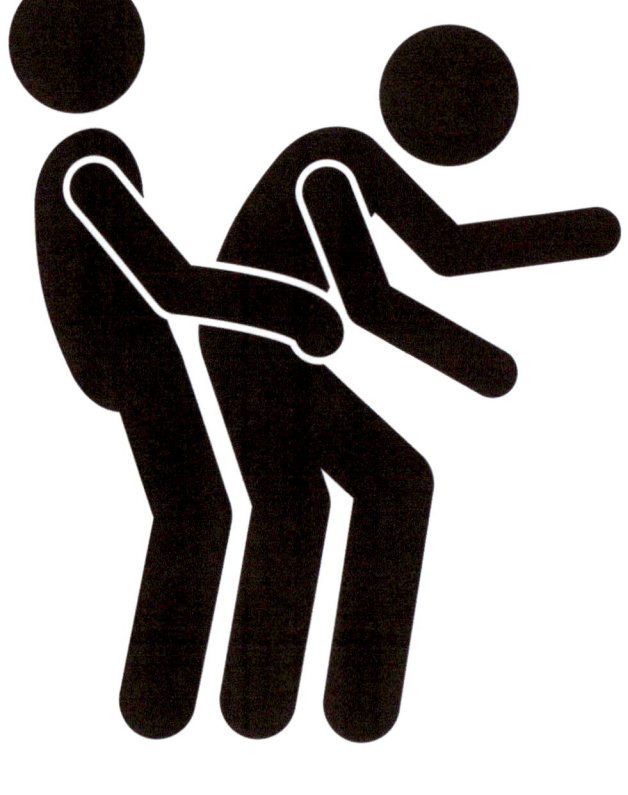

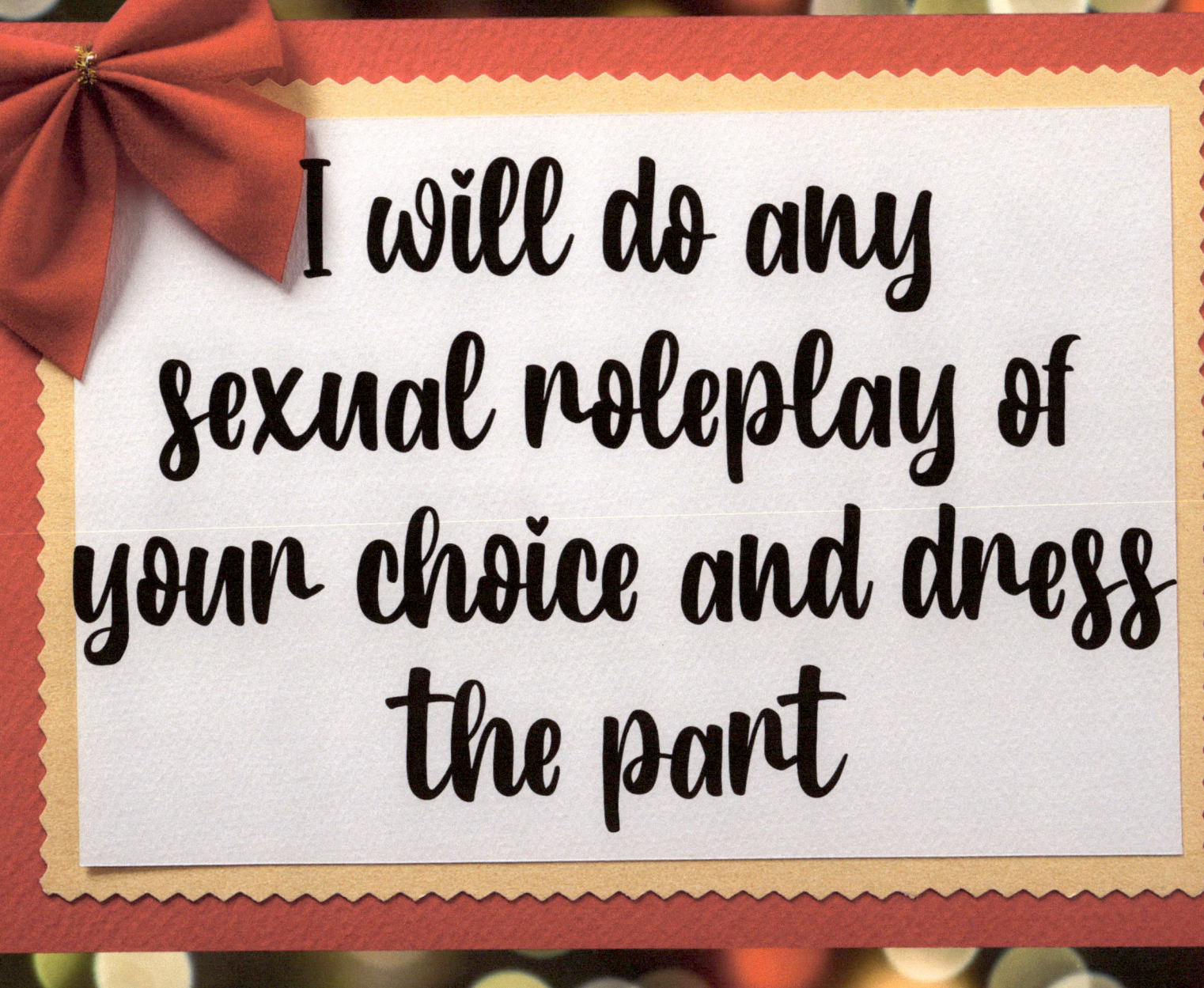

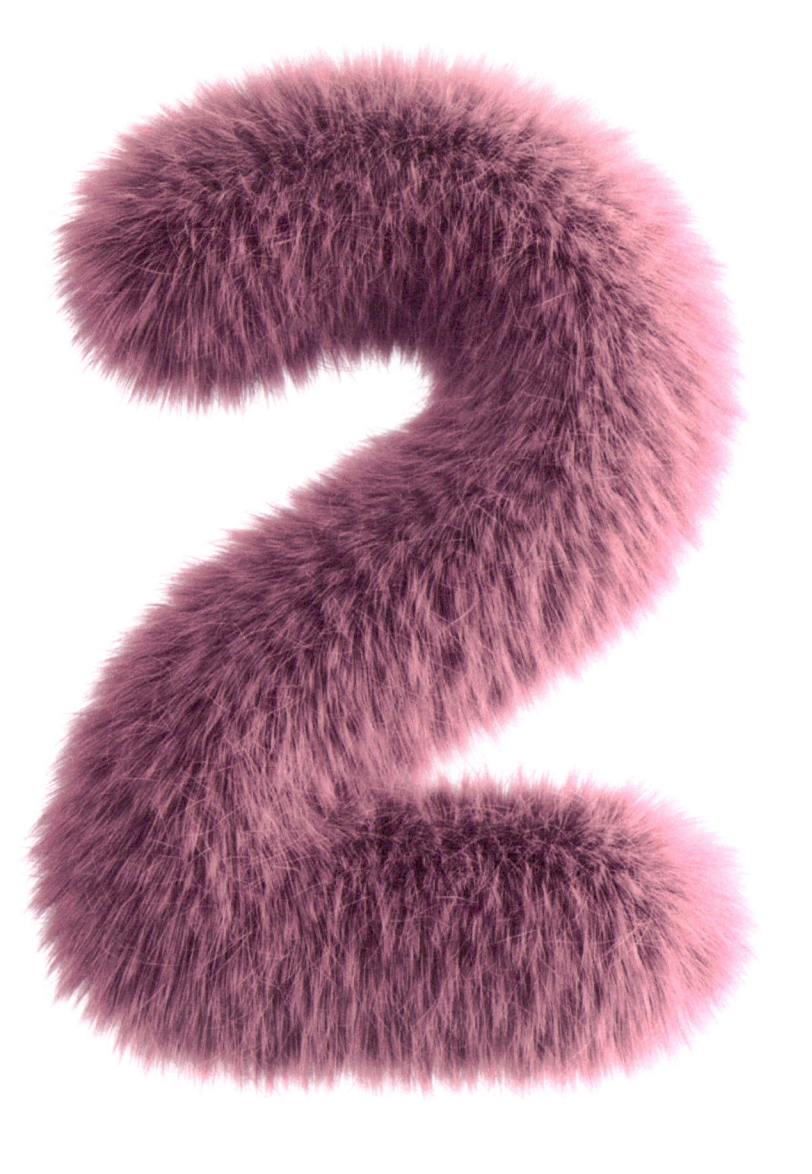 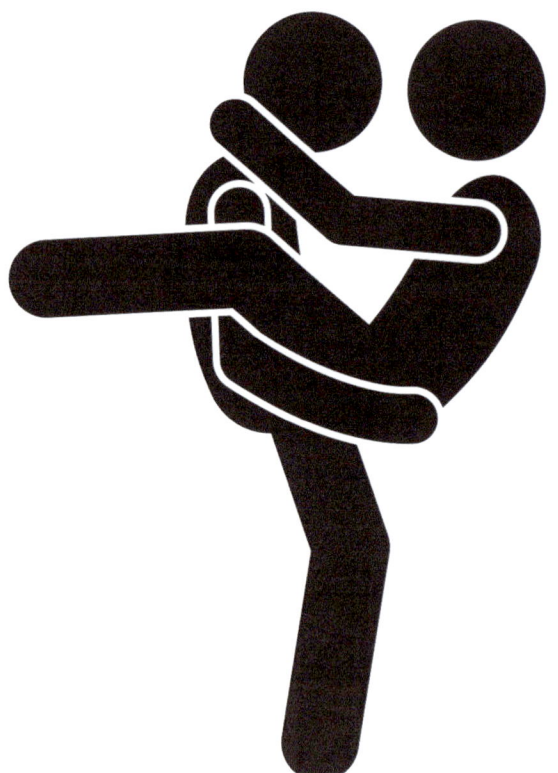

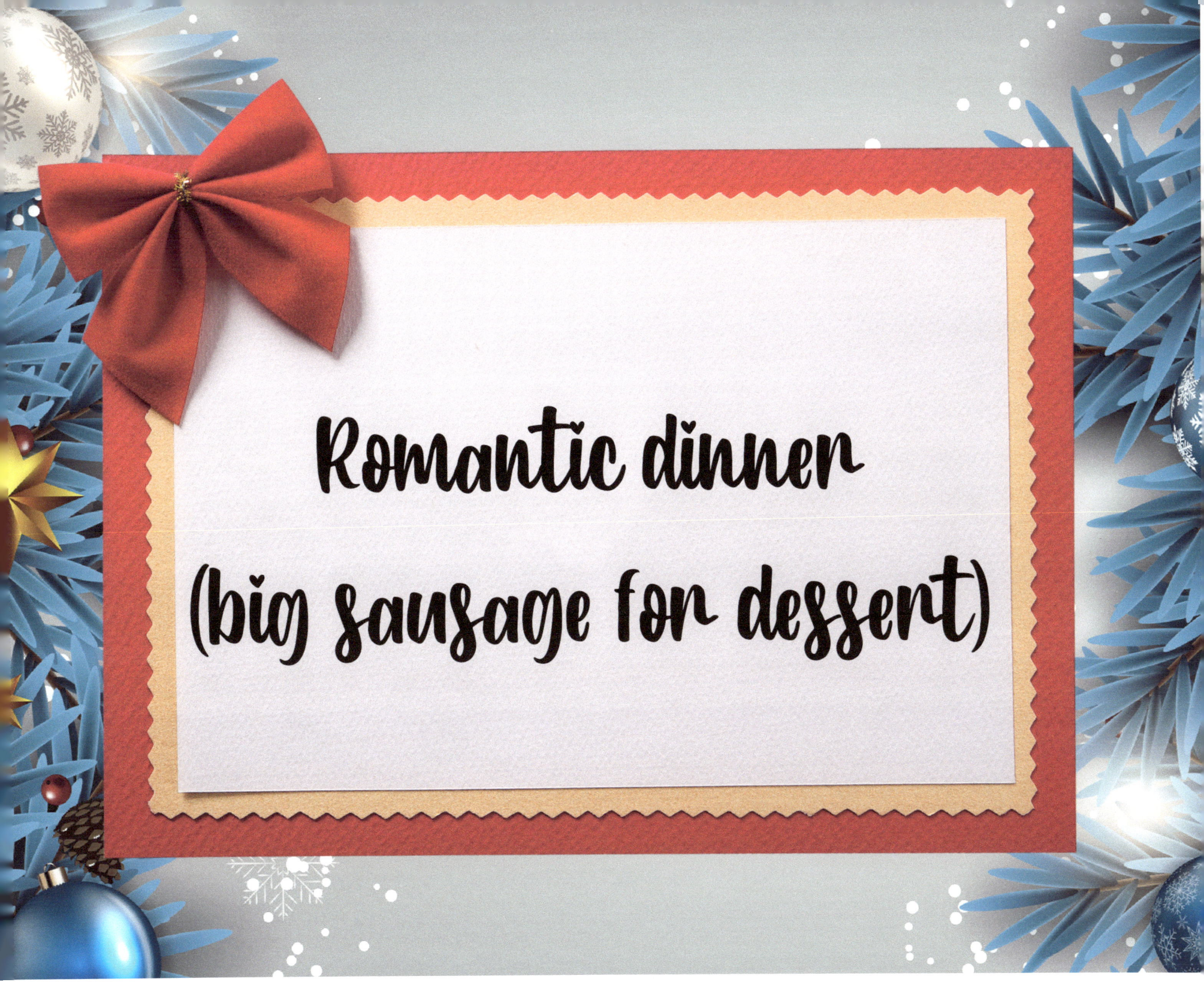

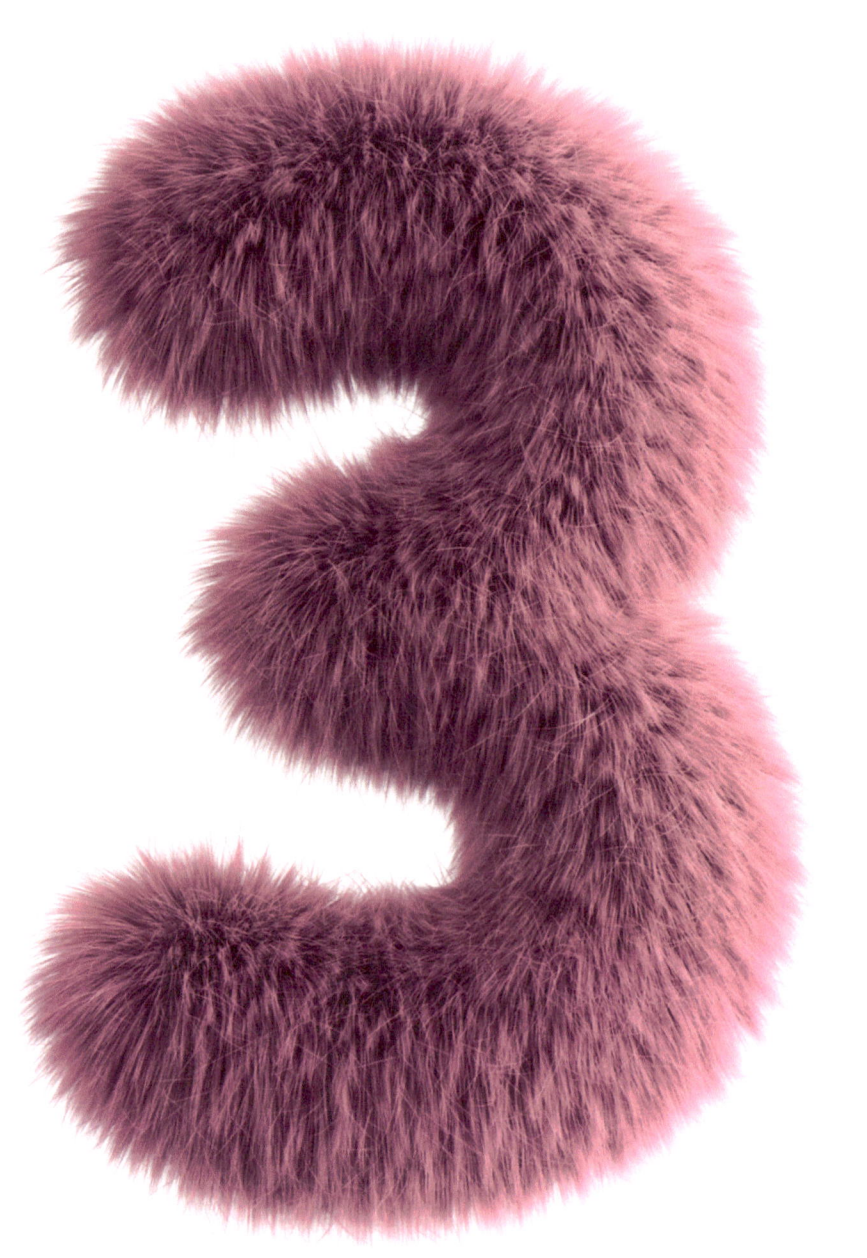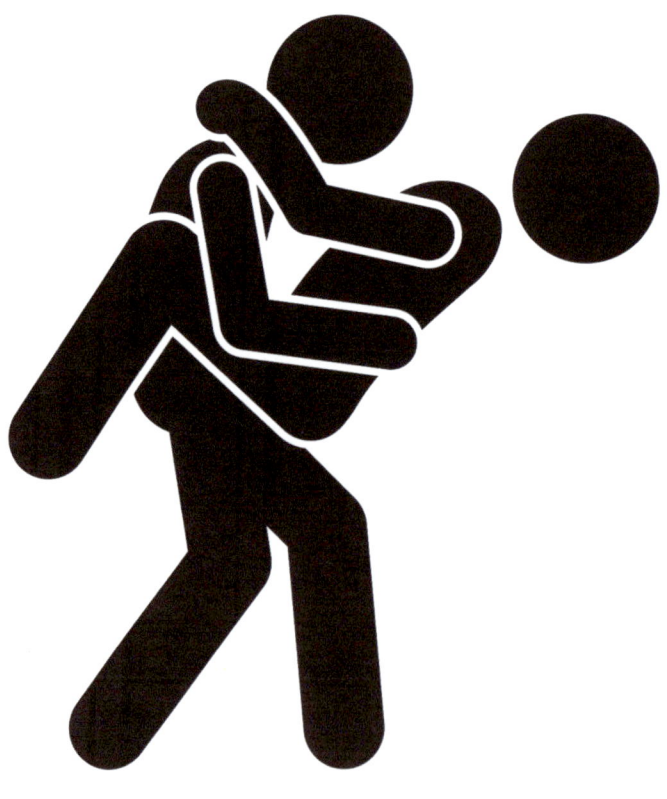

I will pamper you. Face mask, bath, nails done etc

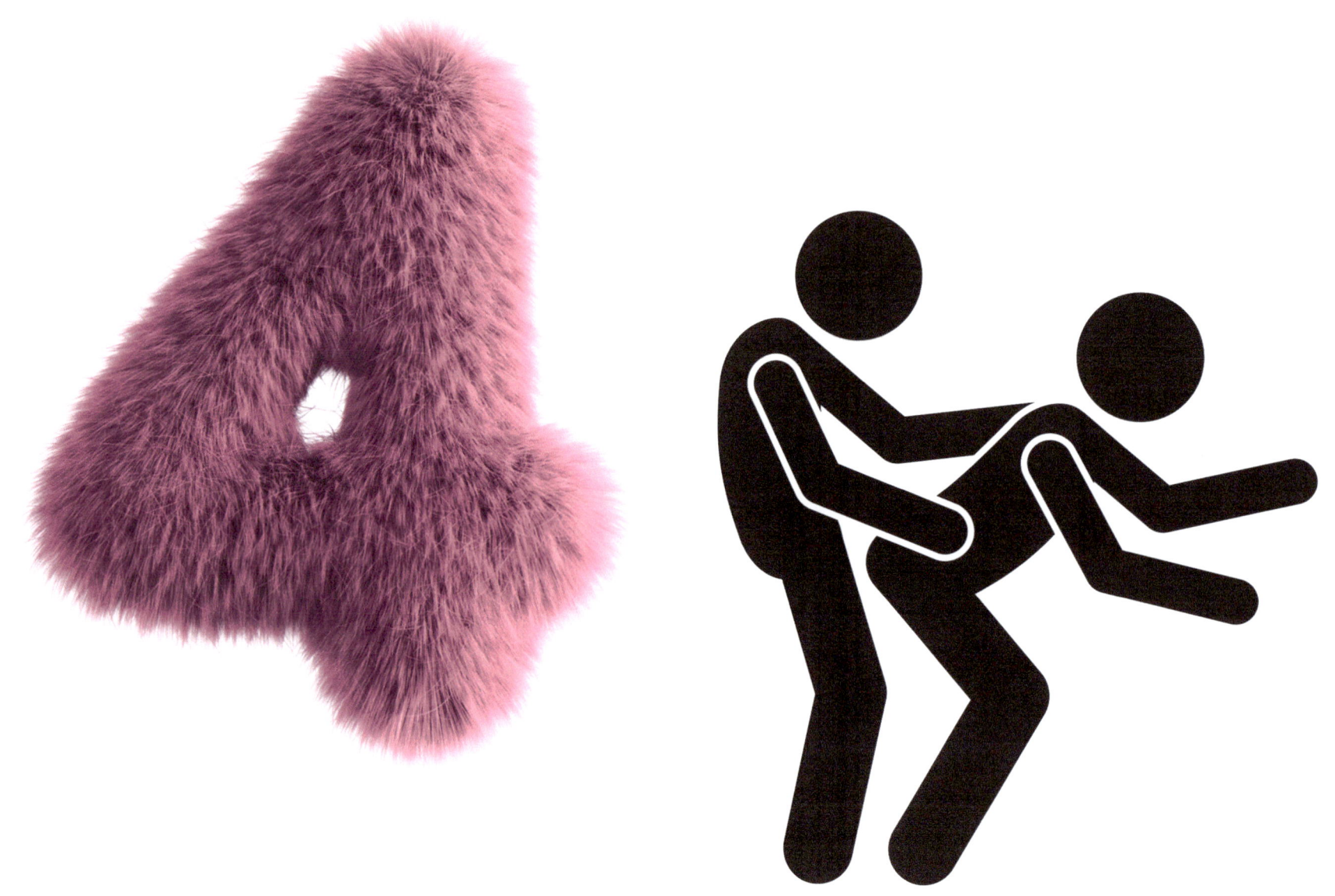

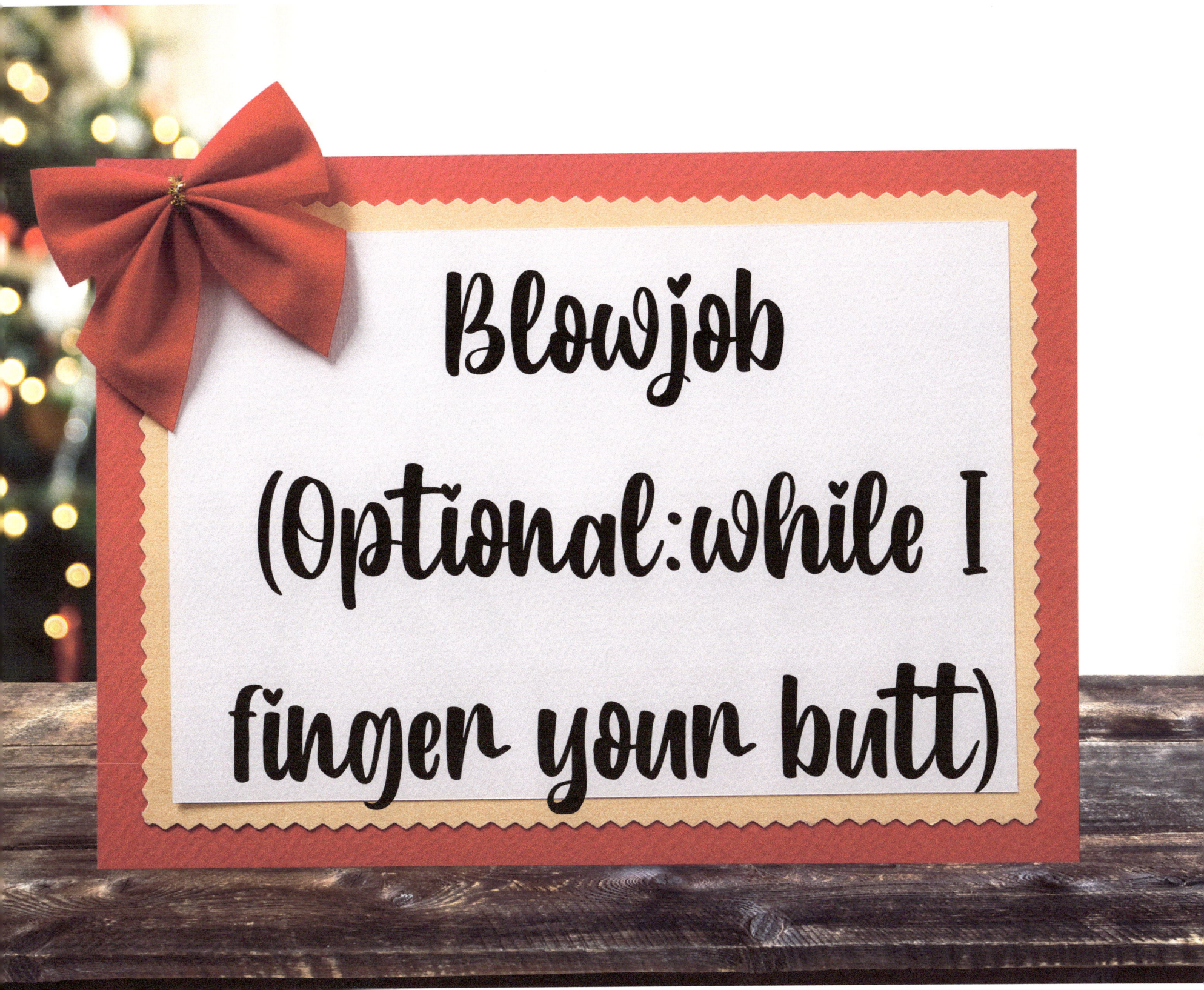

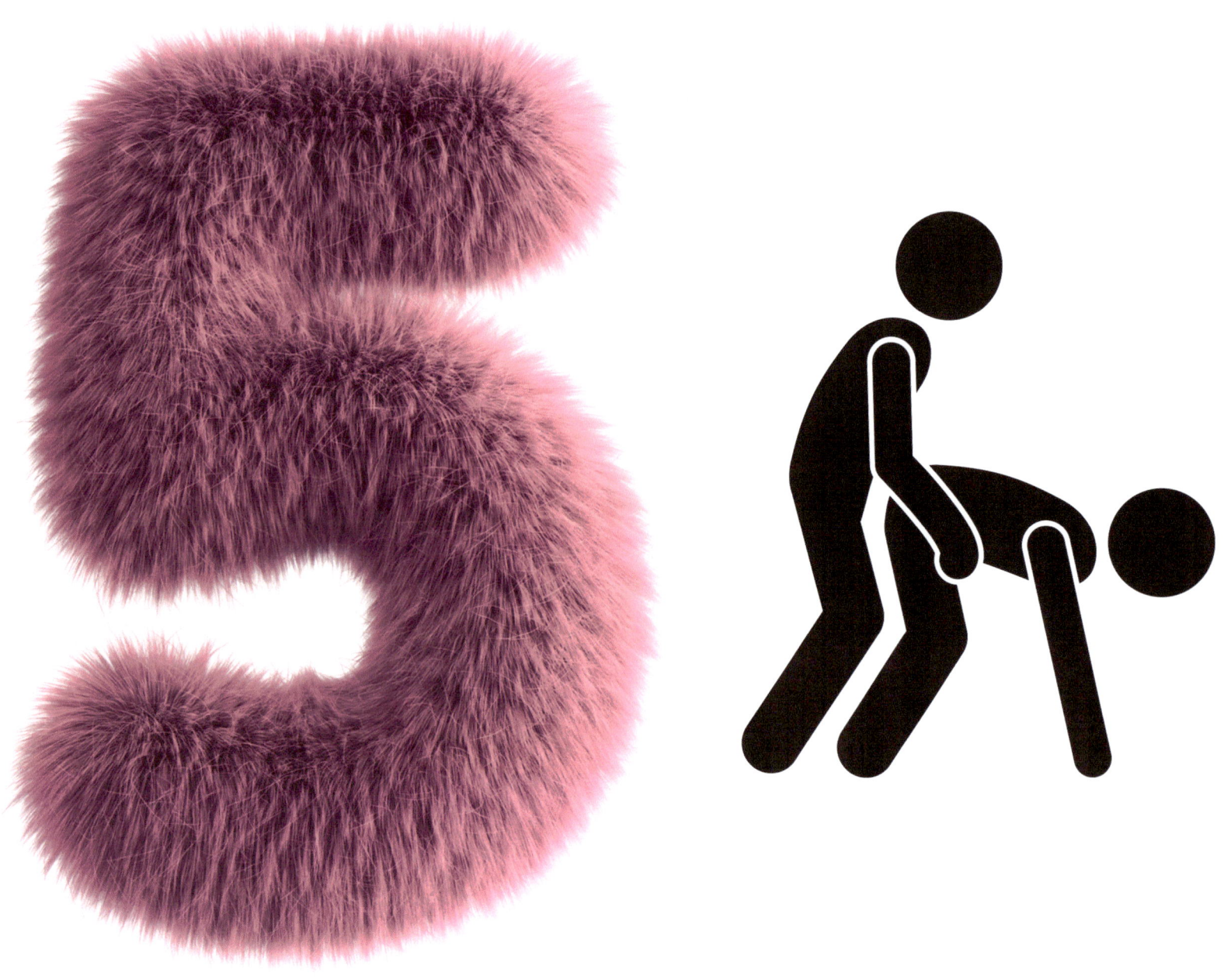

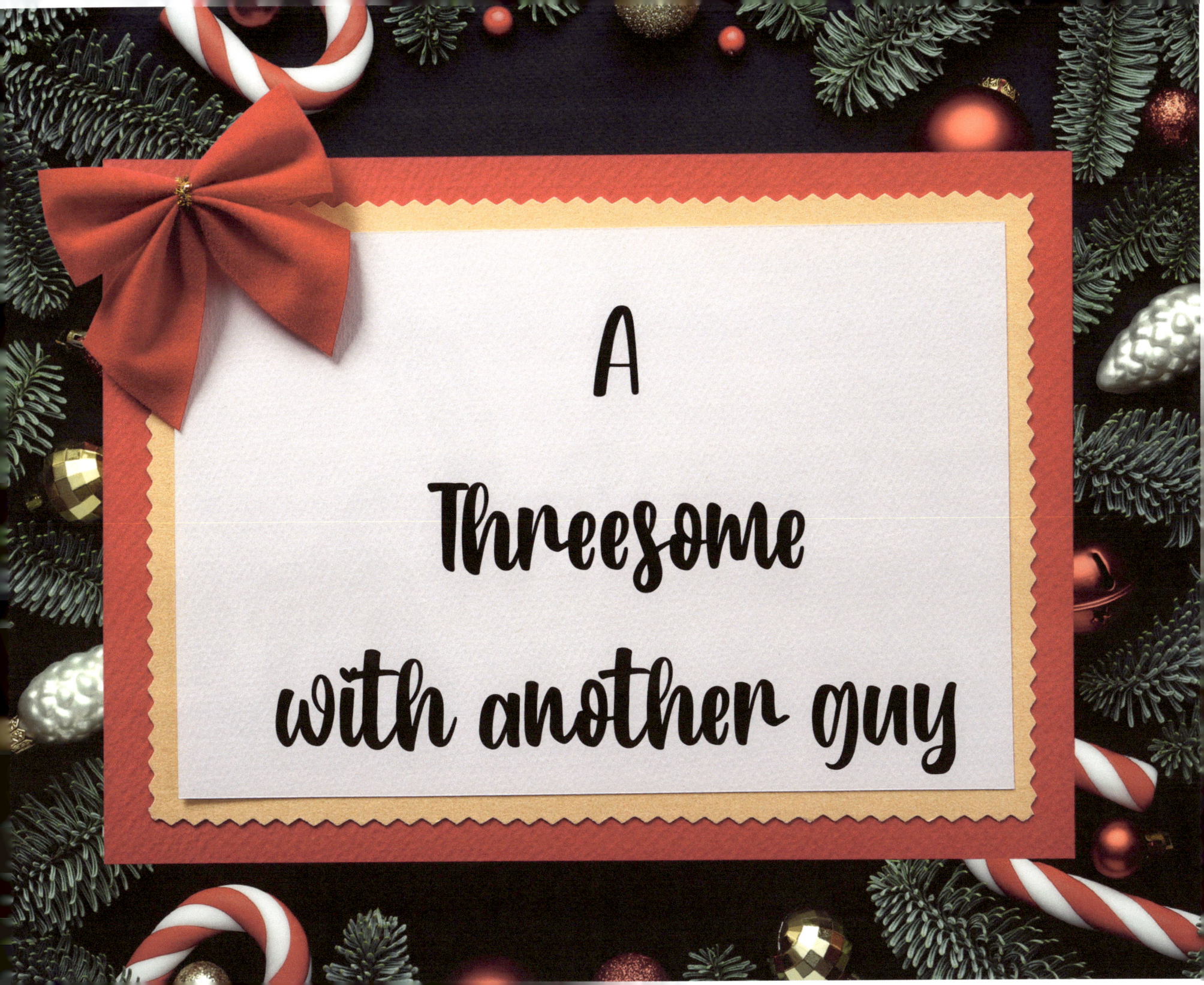

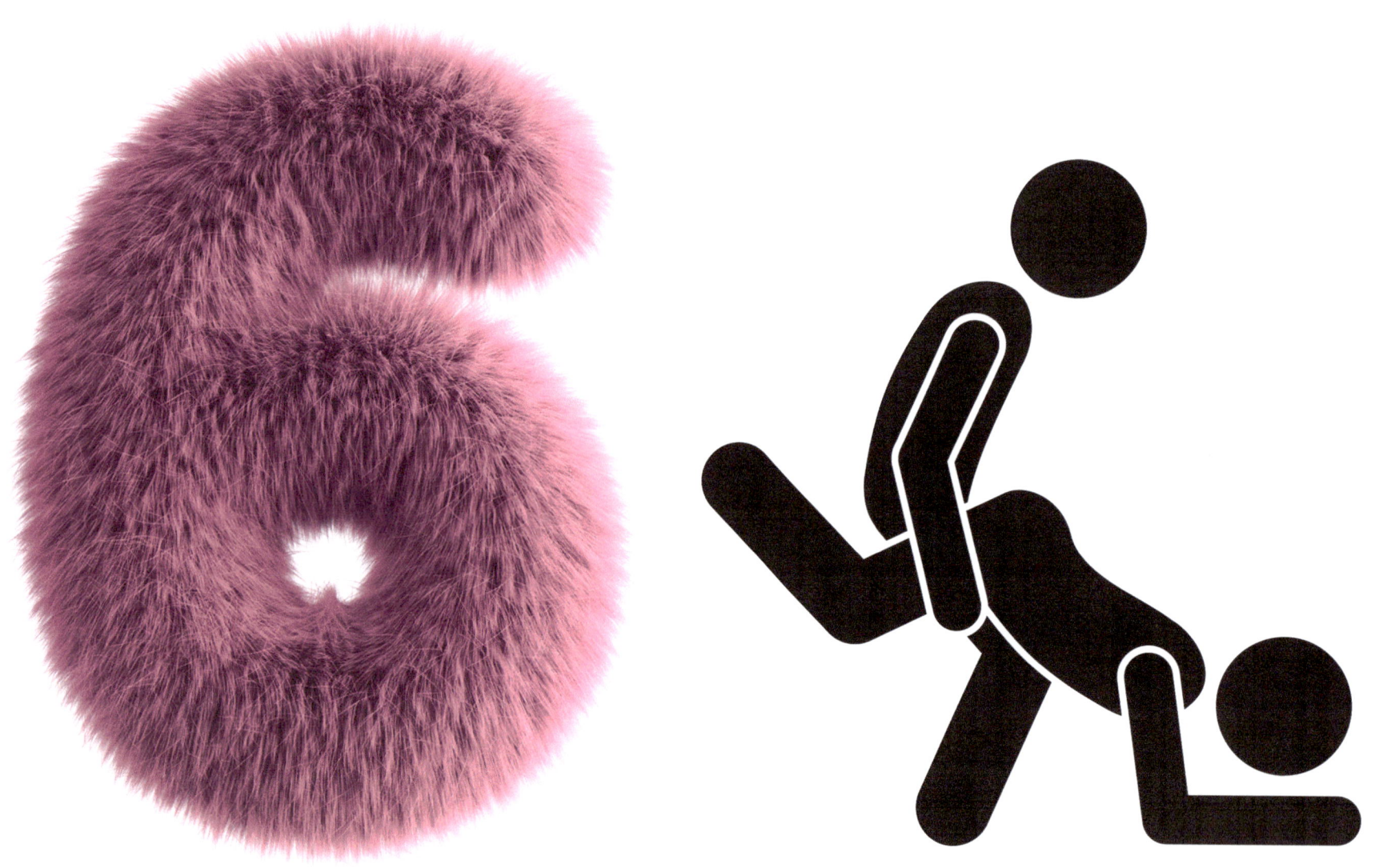

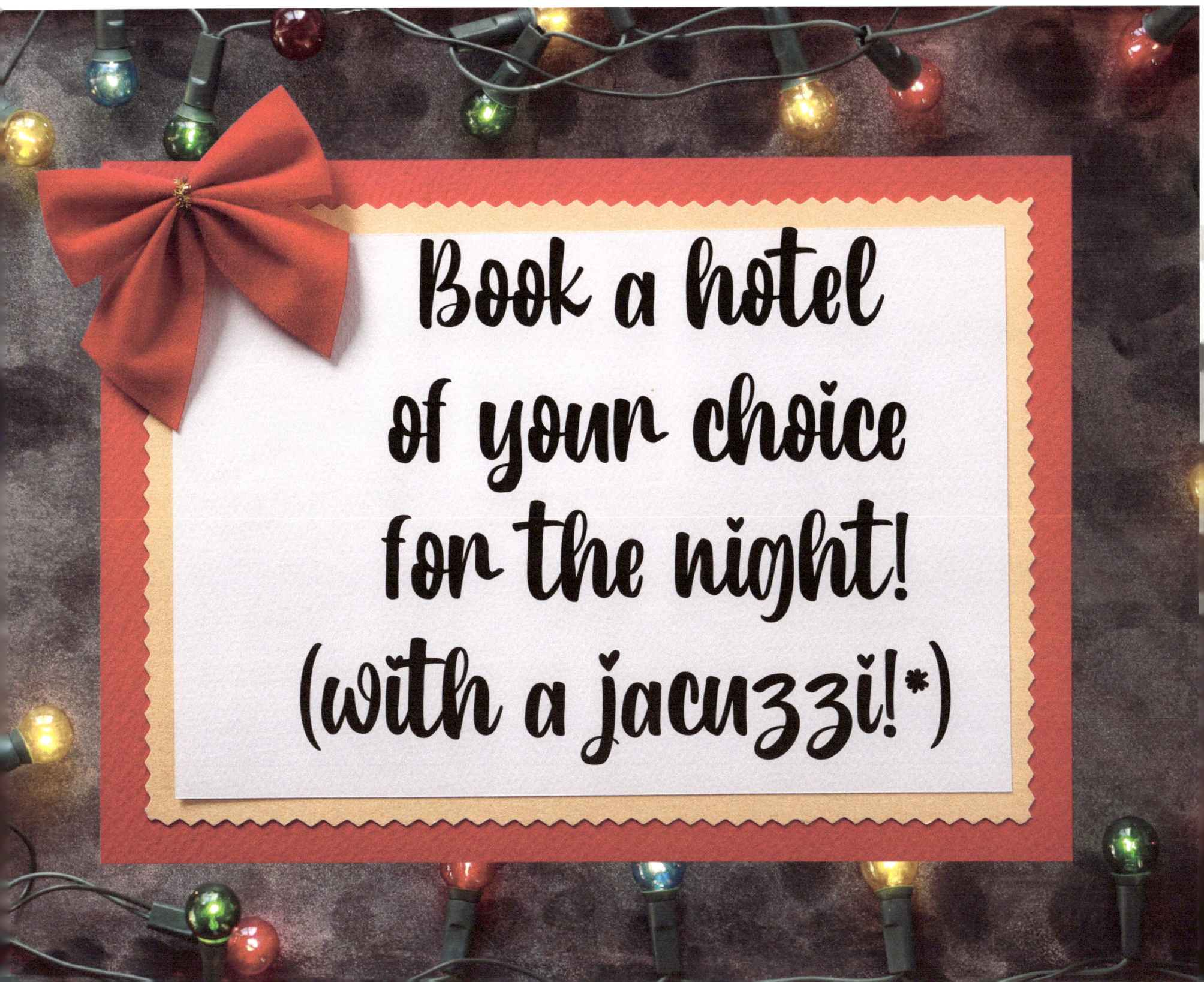

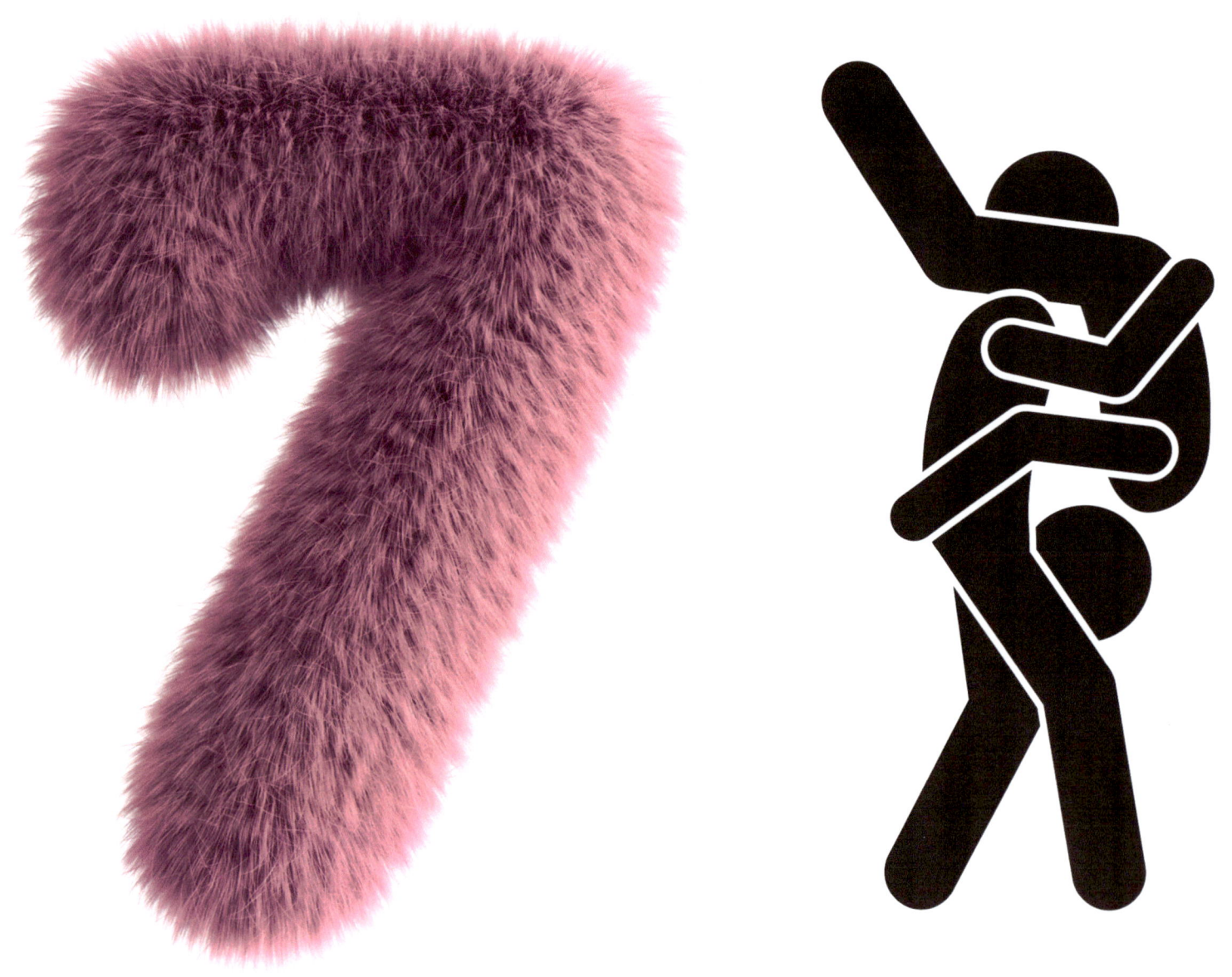

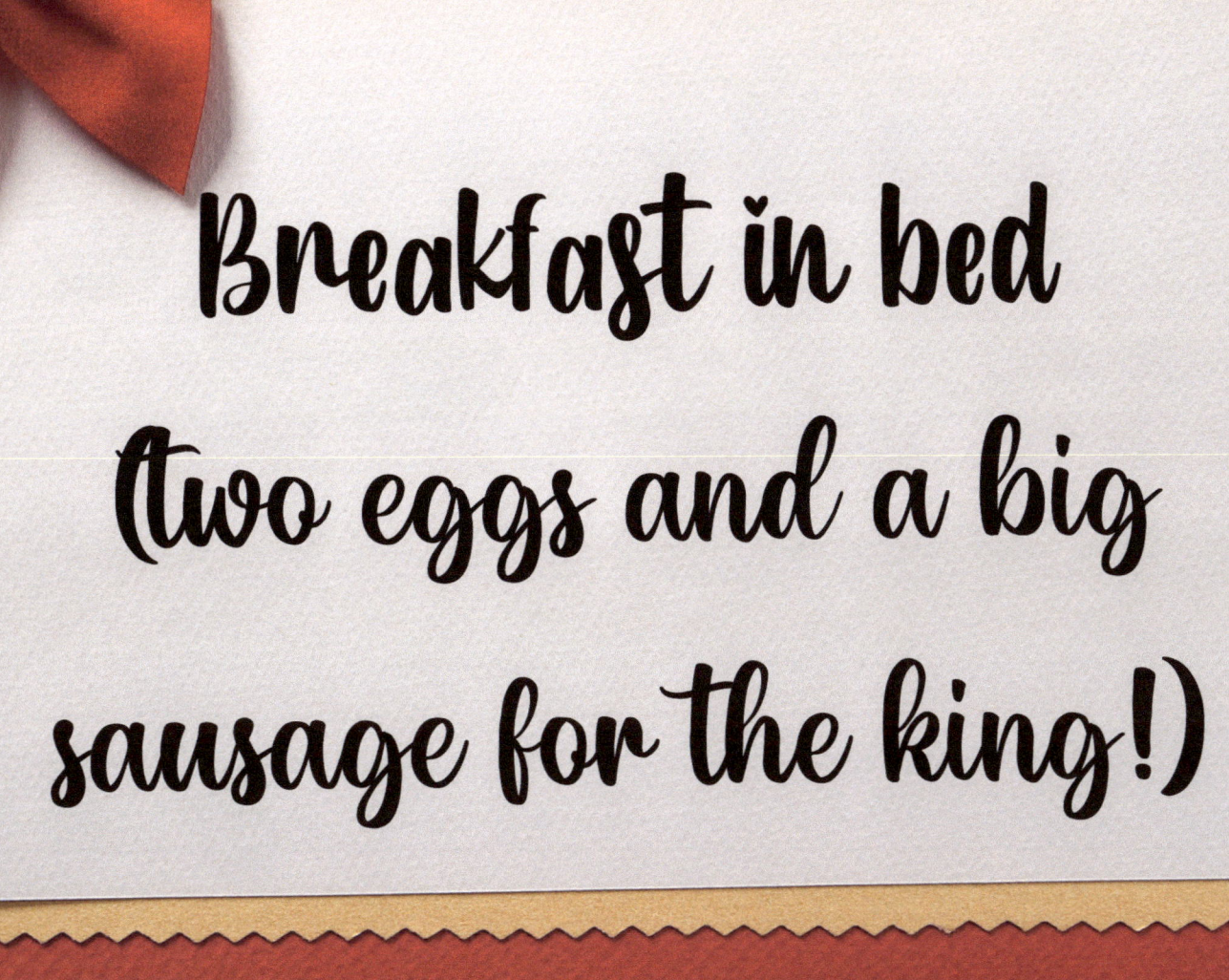

Breakfast in bed (two eggs and a big sausage for the king!)

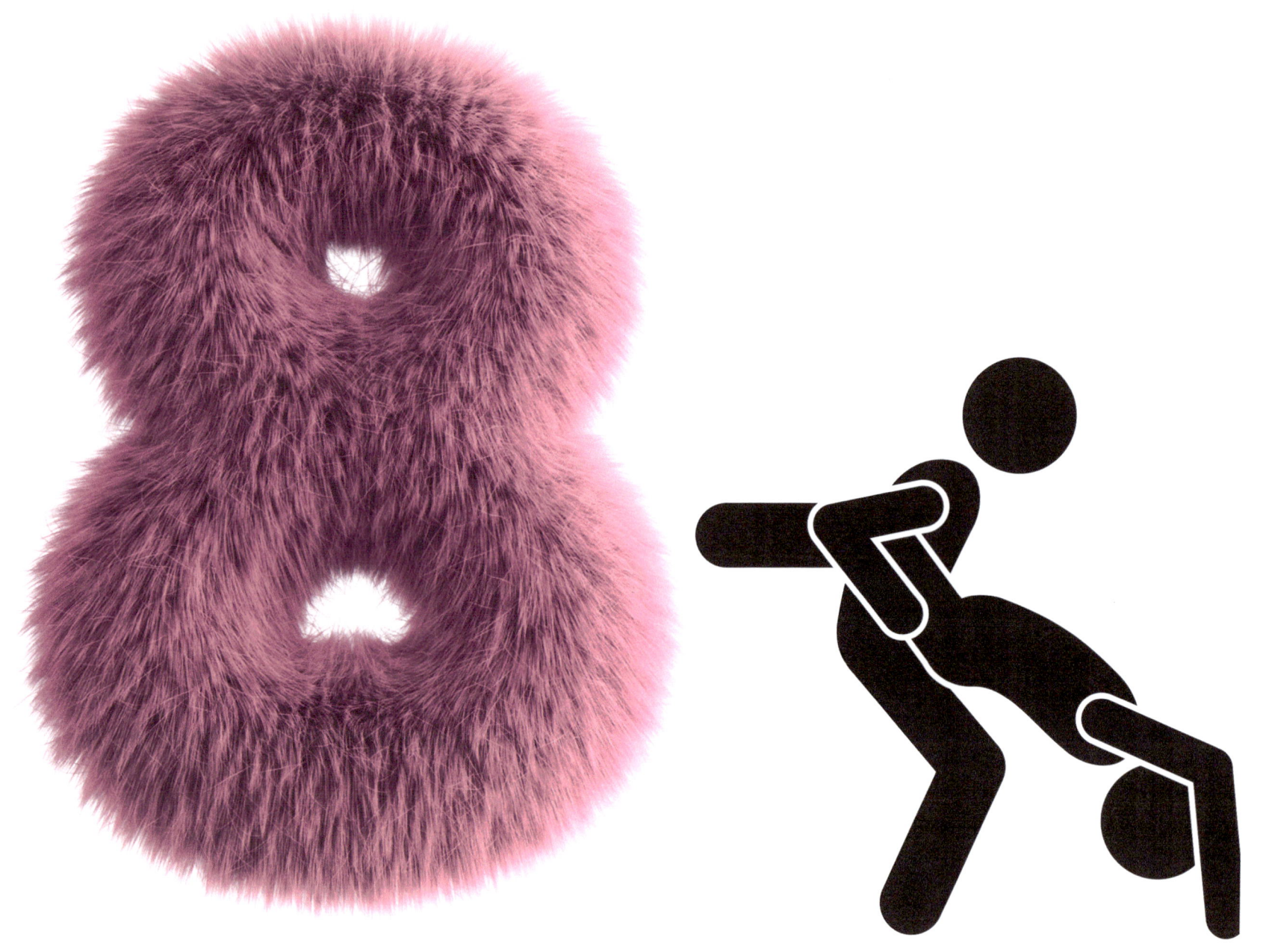

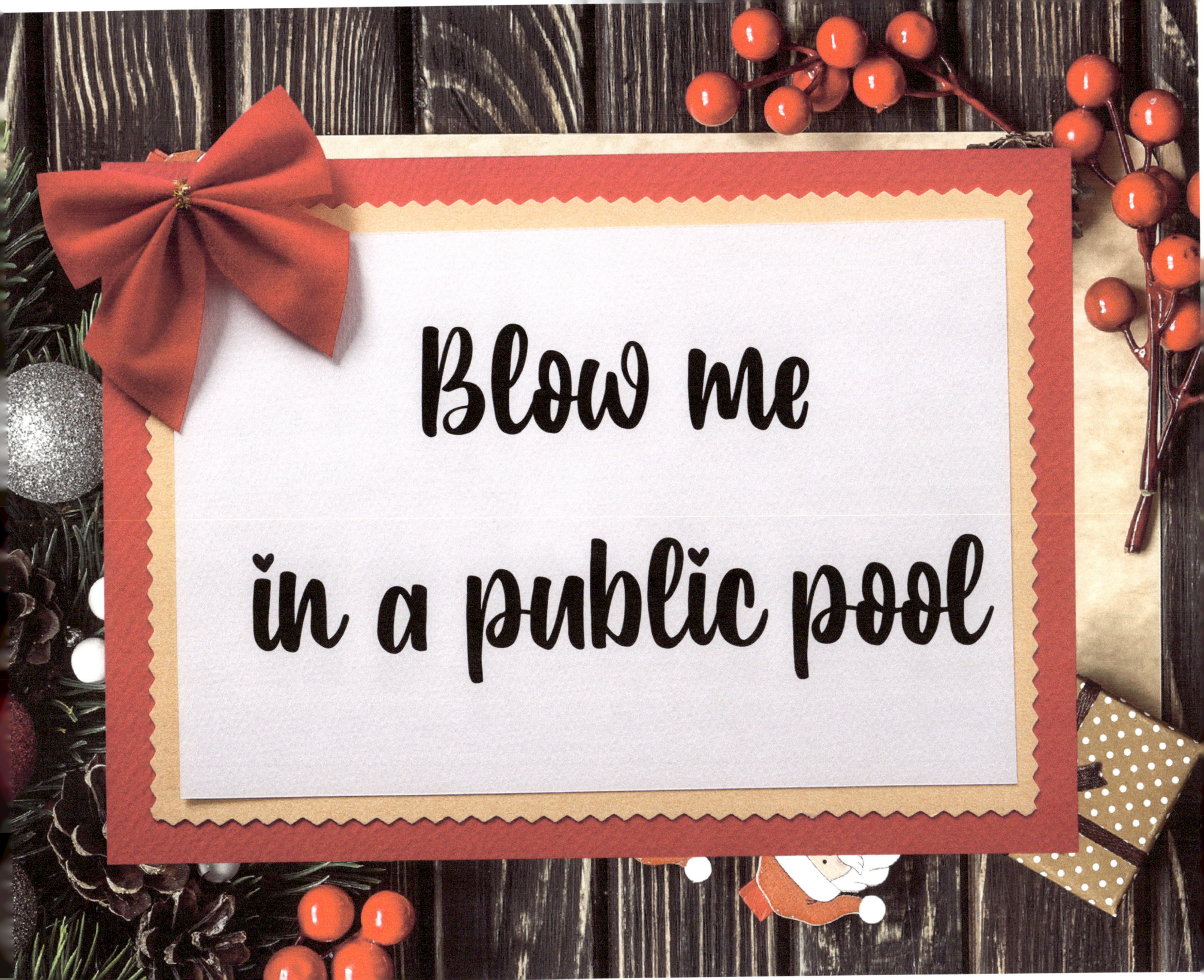

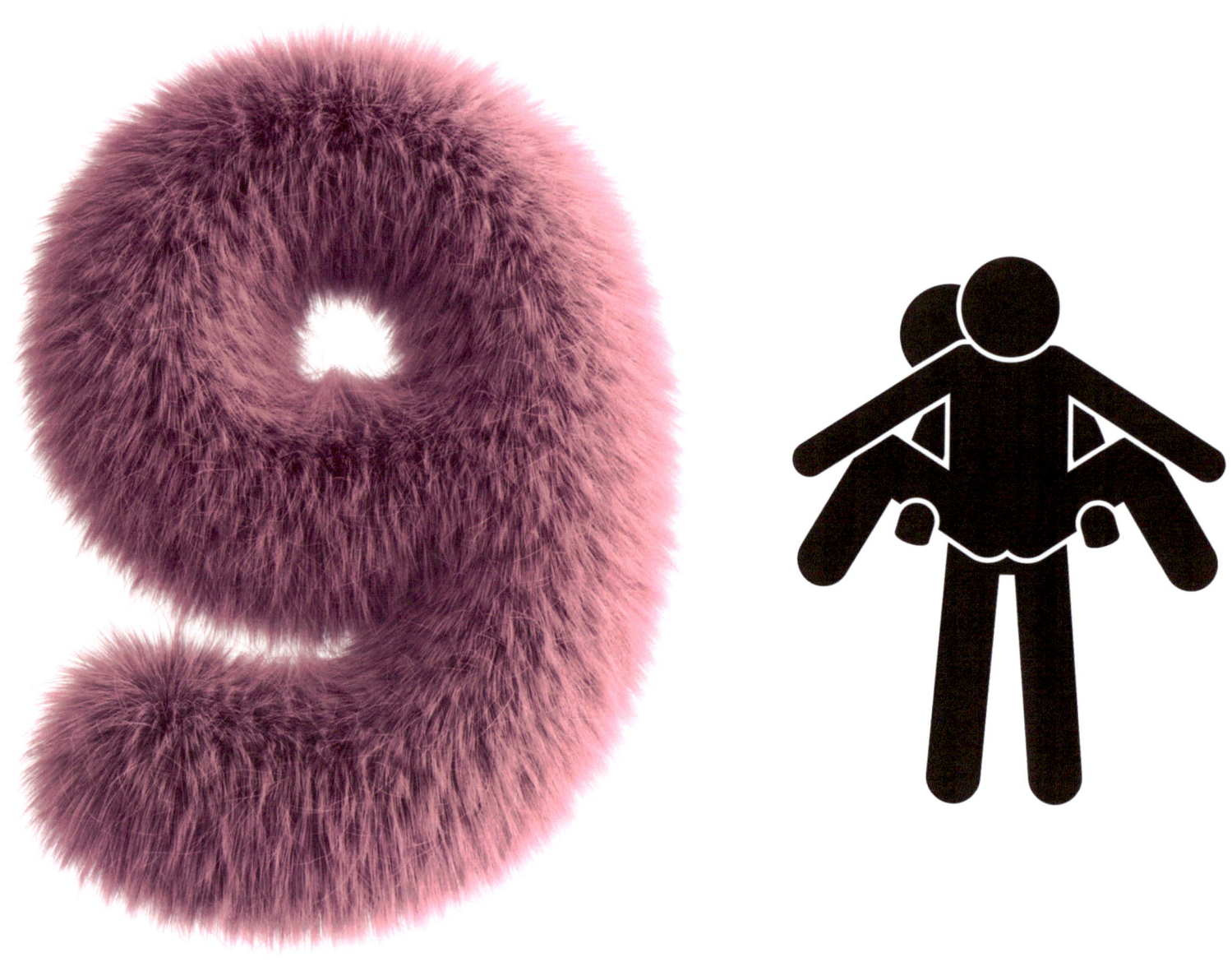

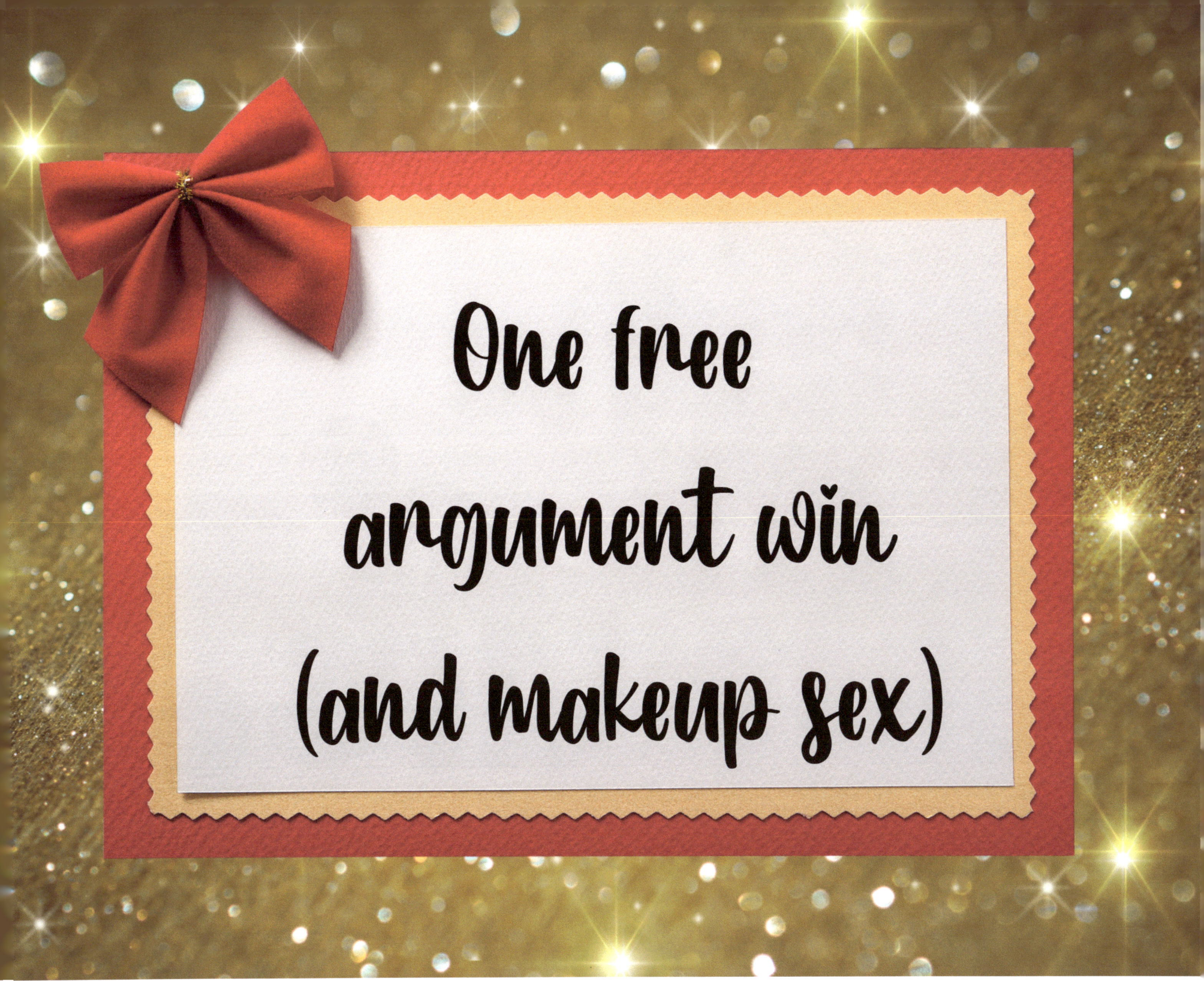

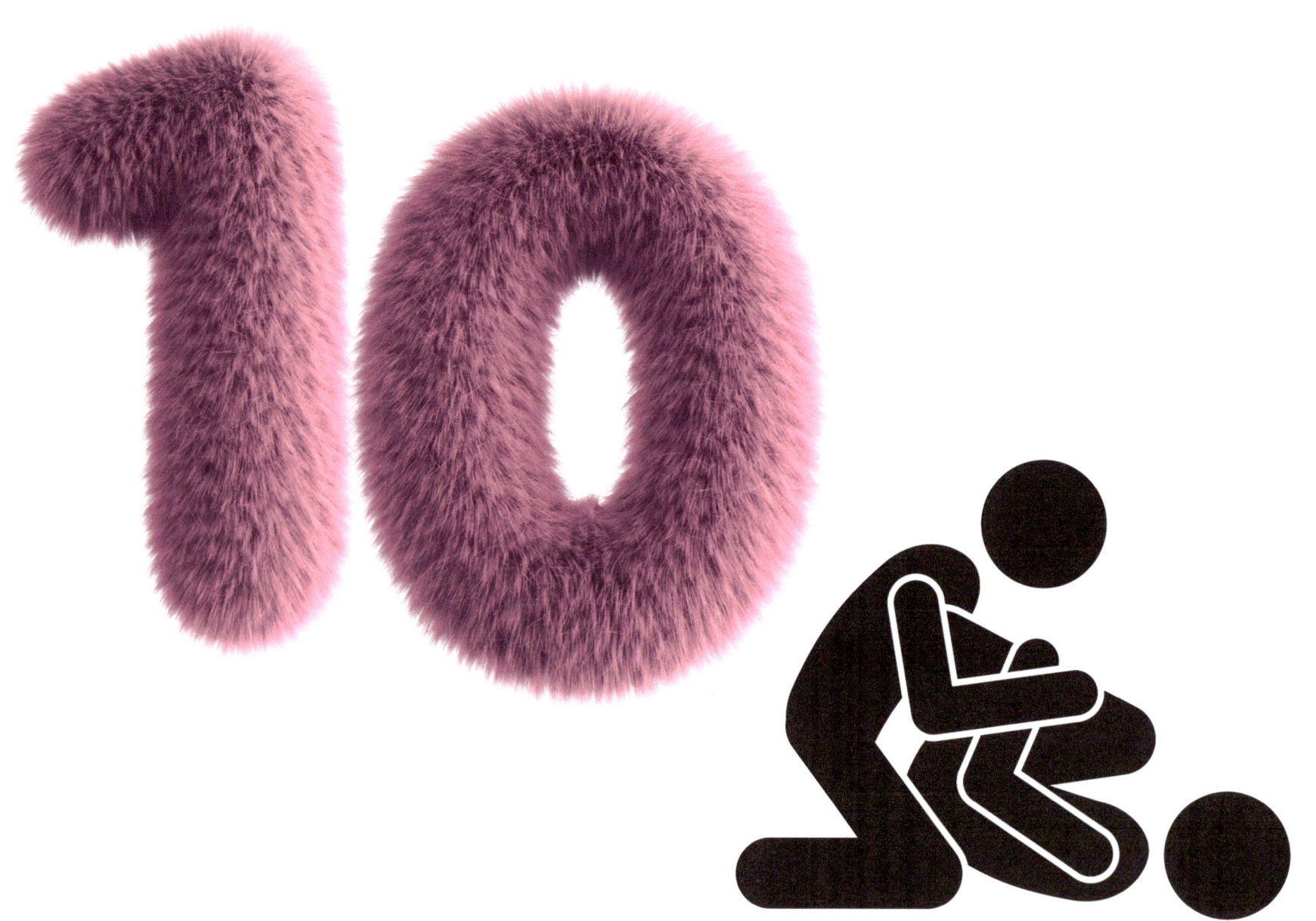

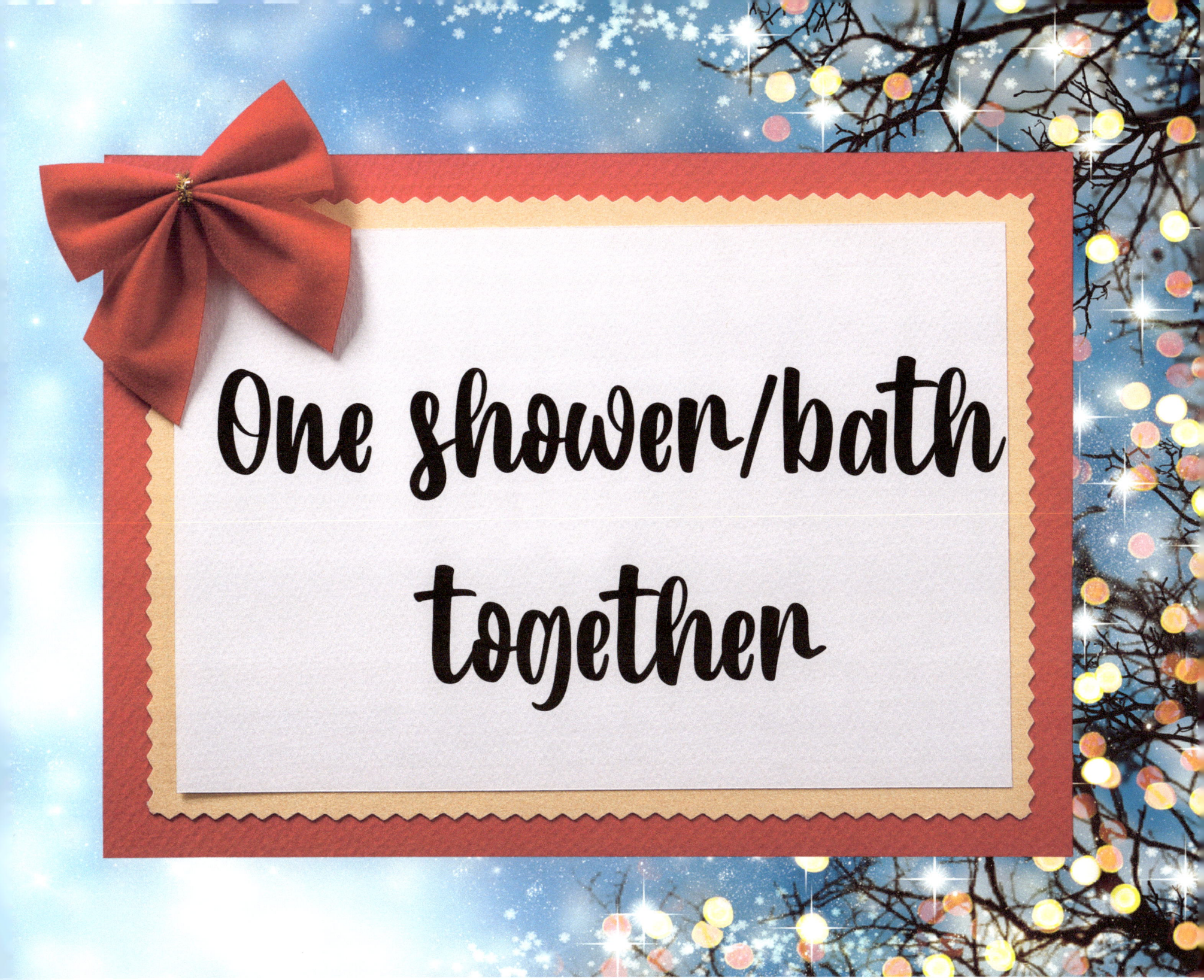

11

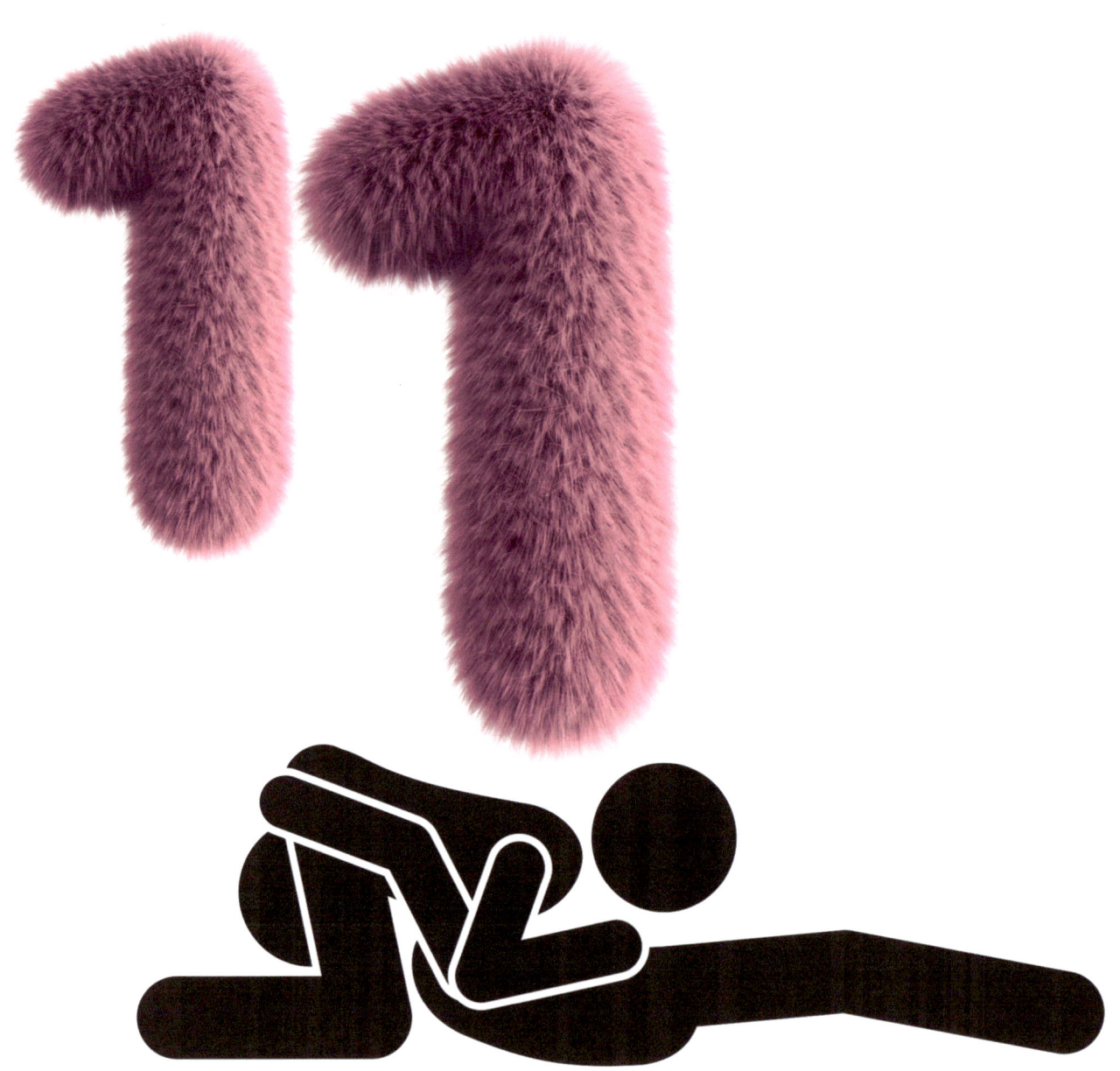

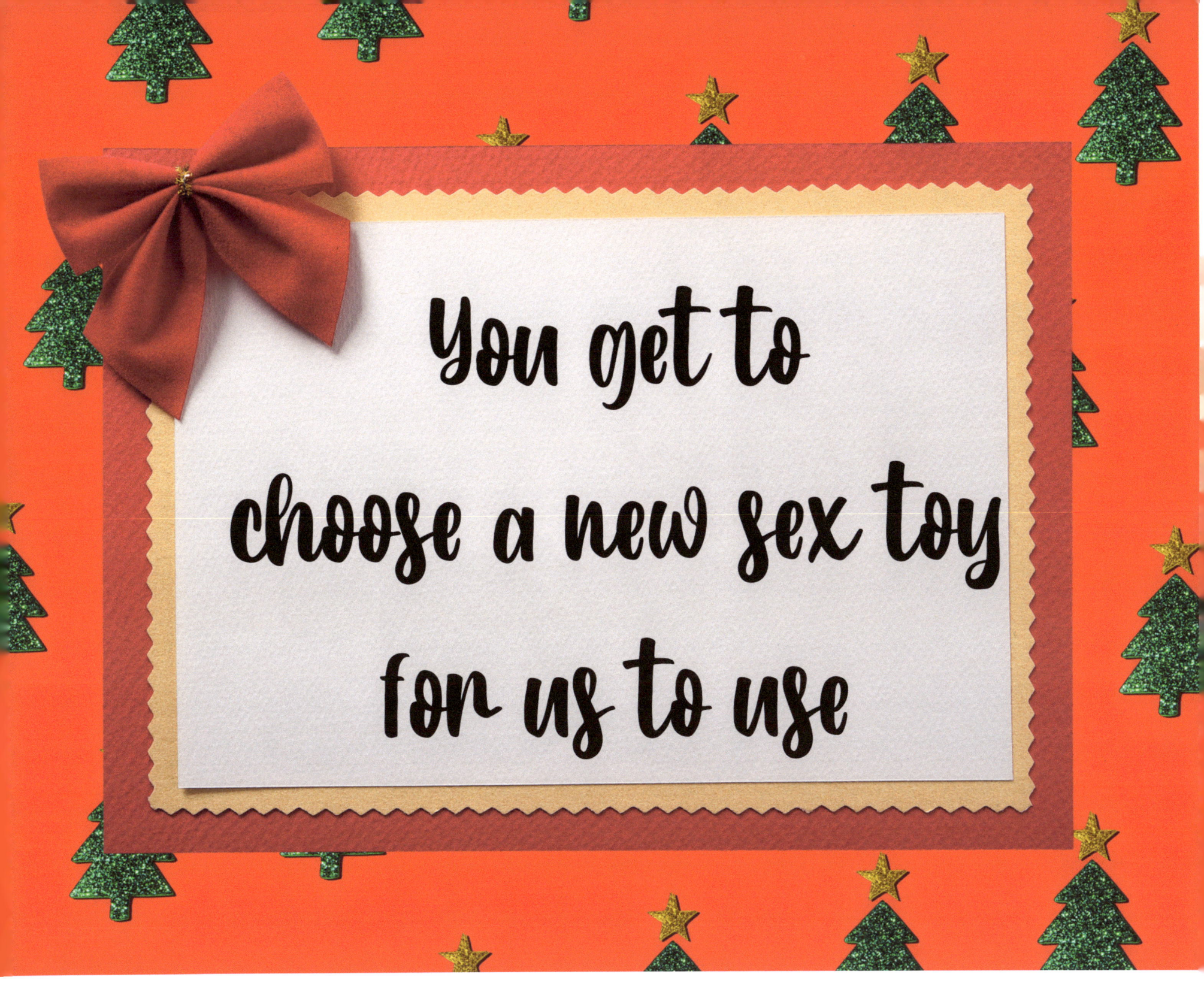

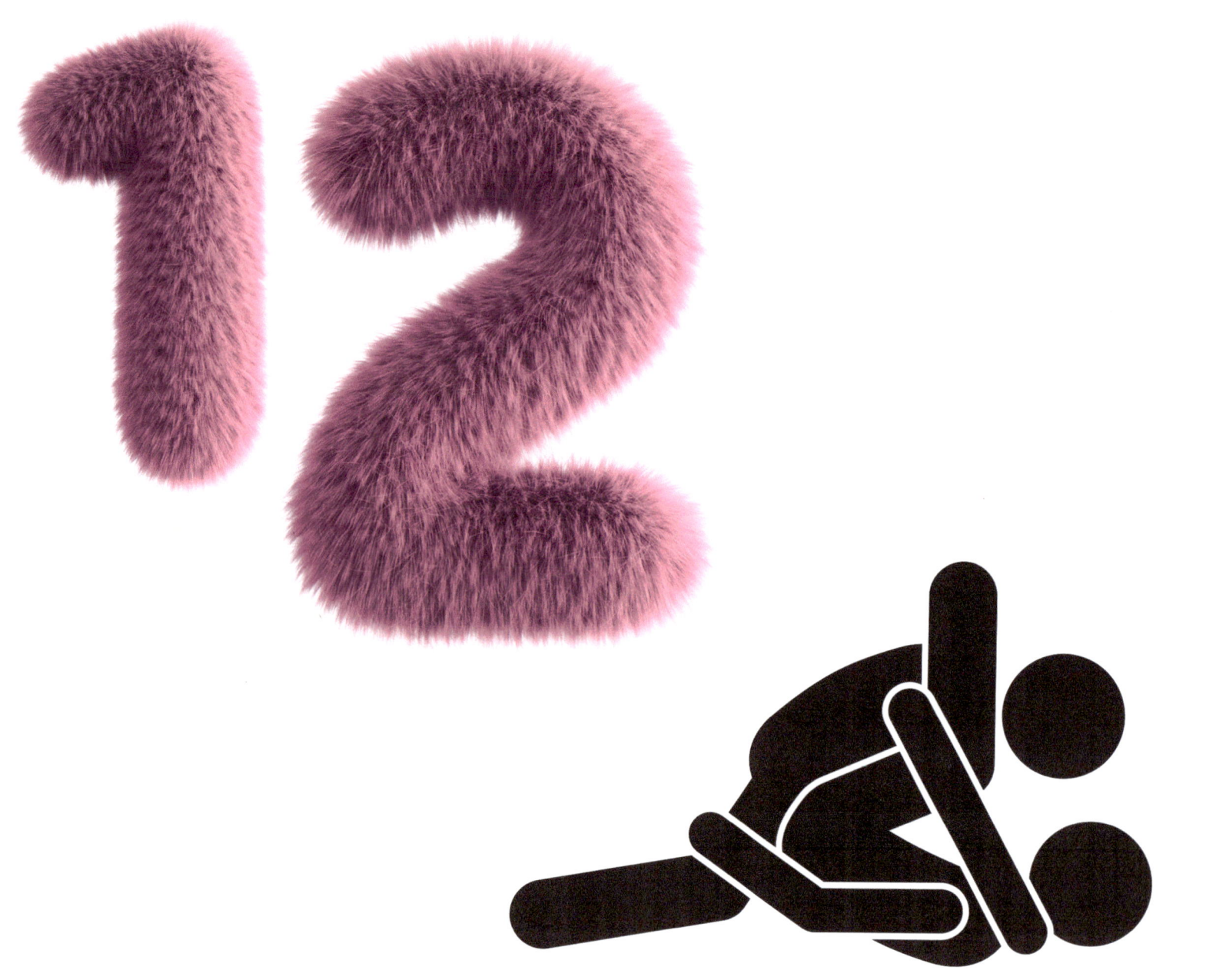

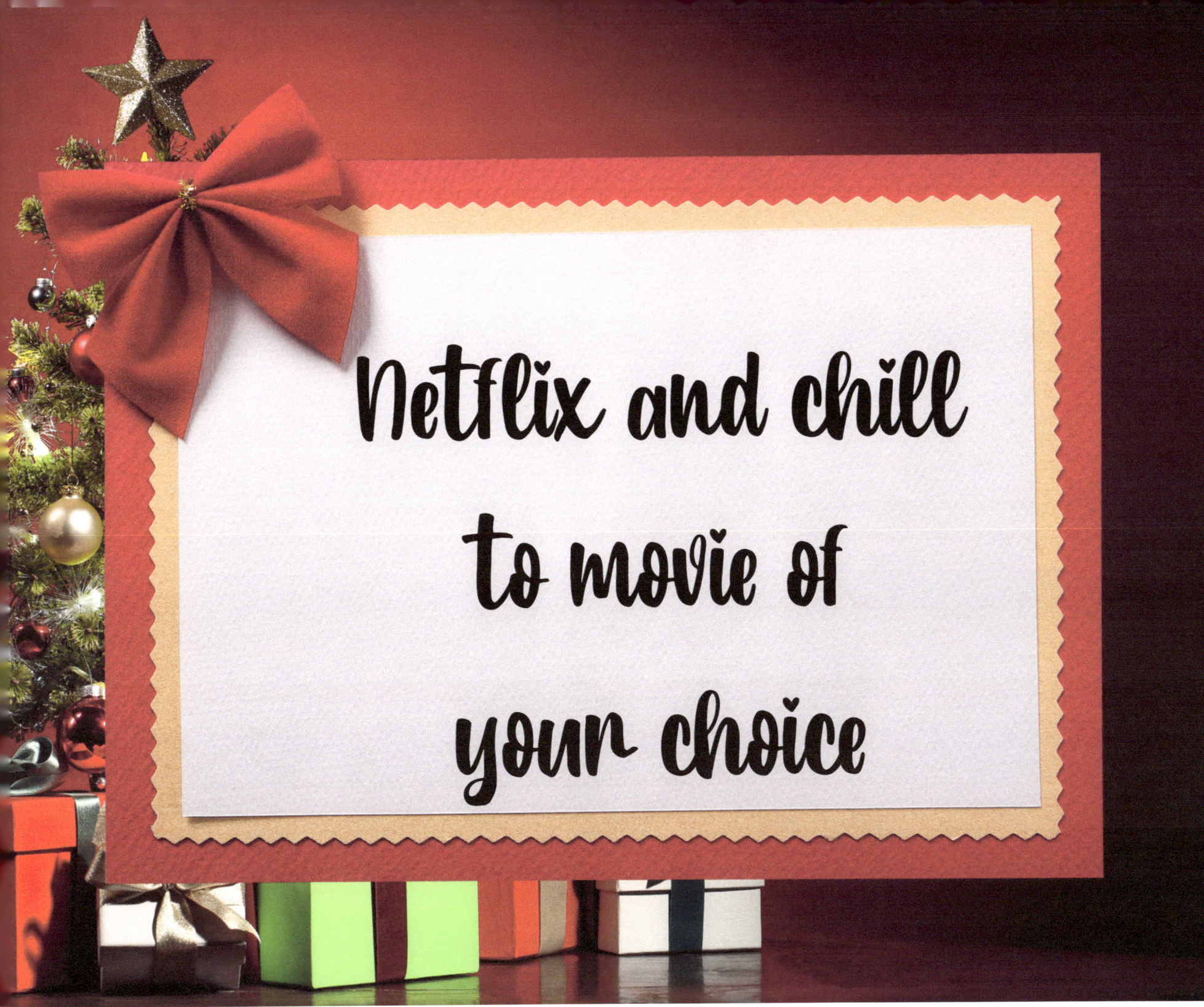

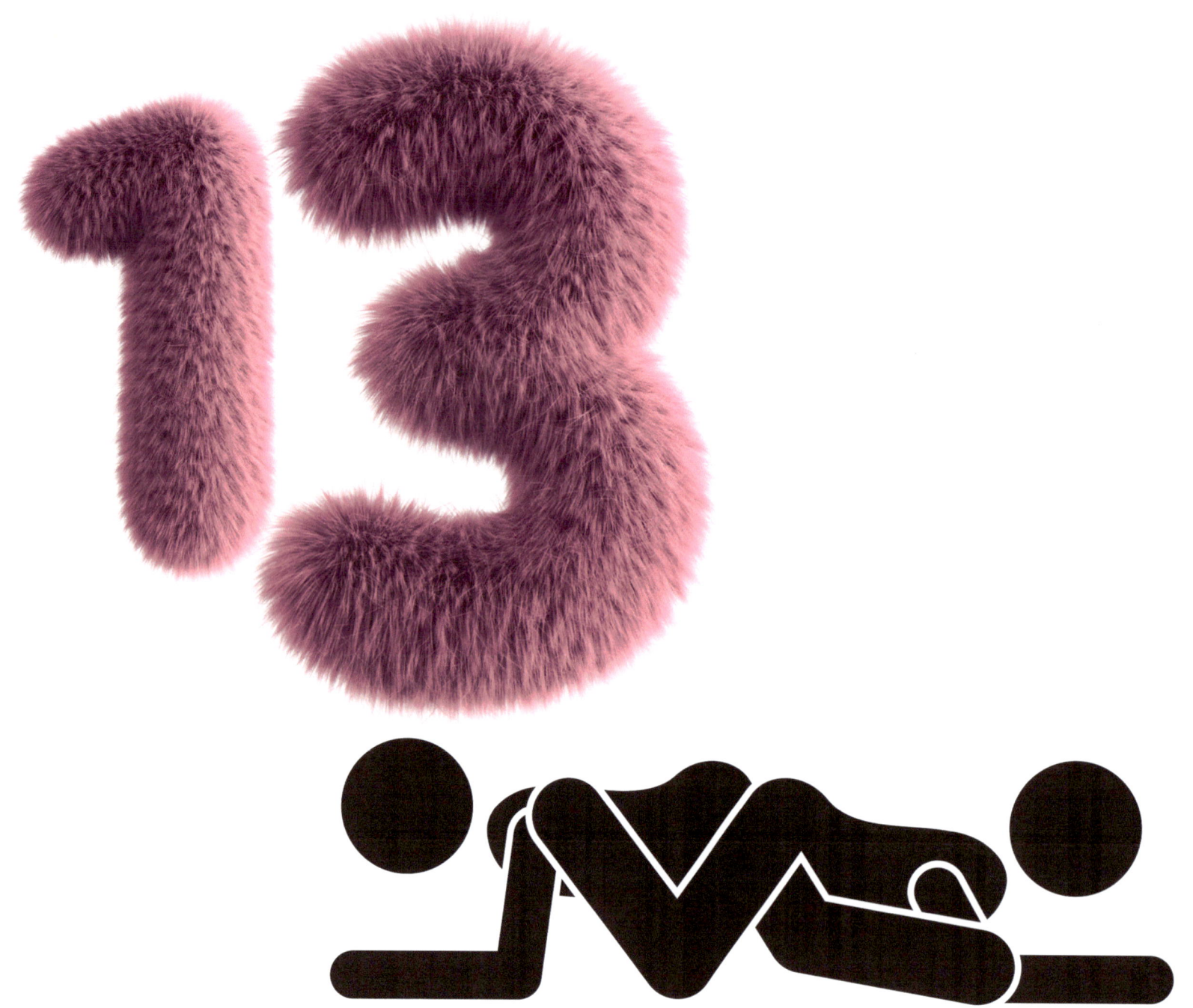

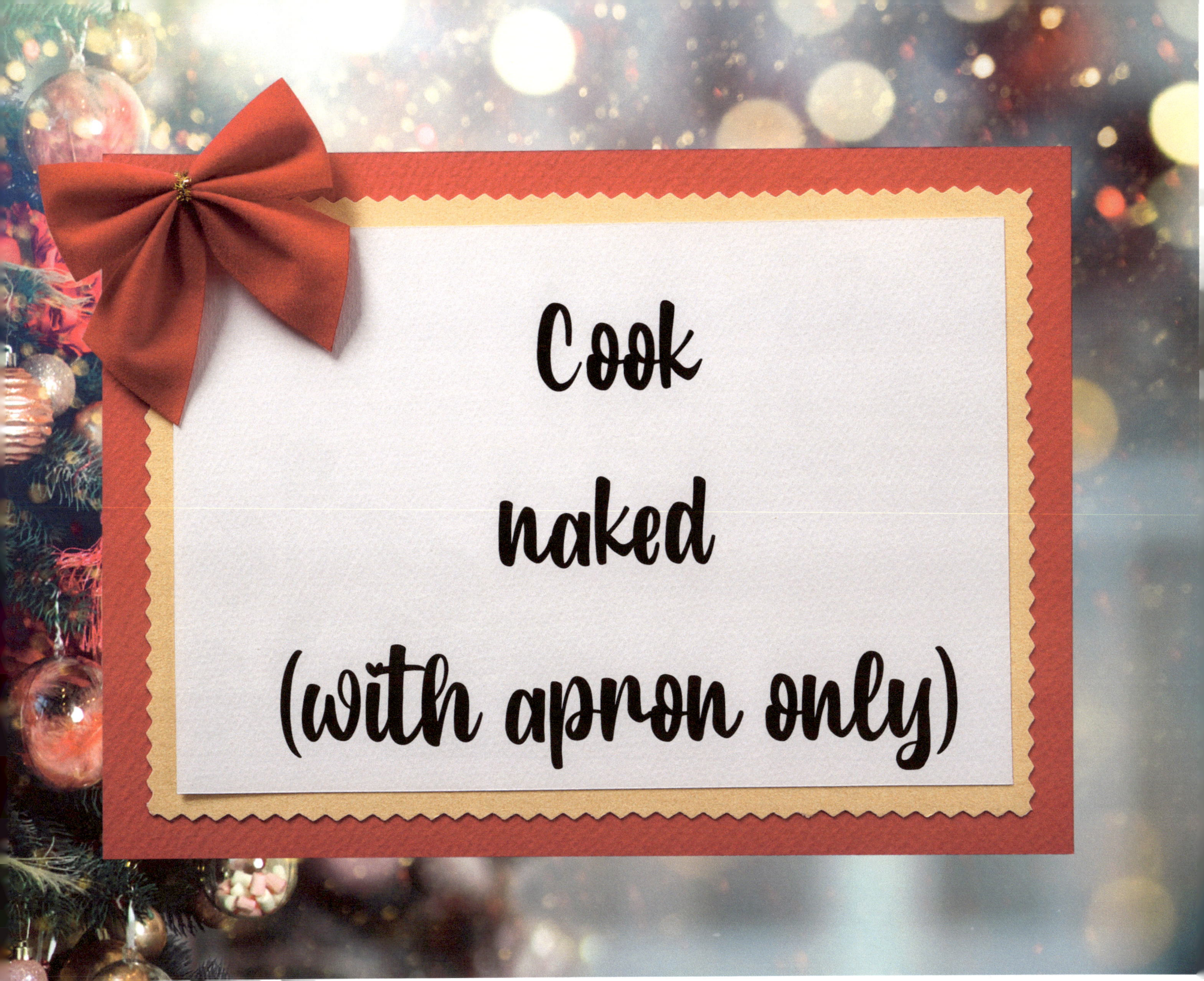

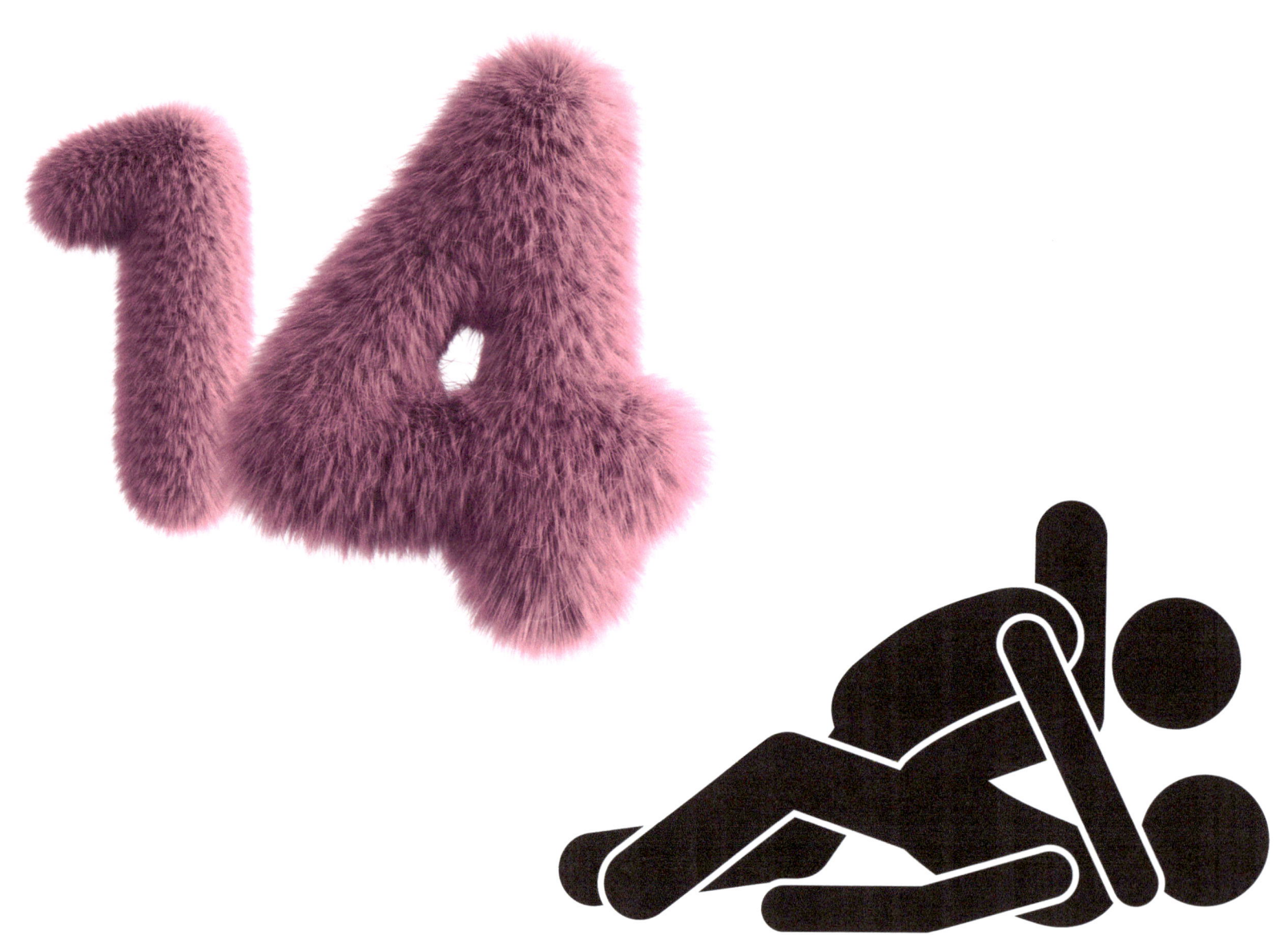

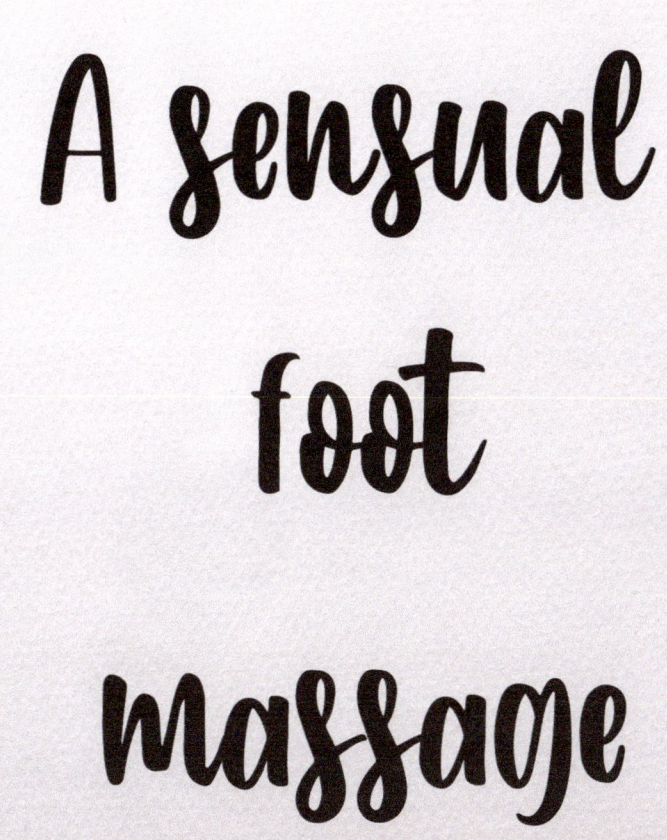

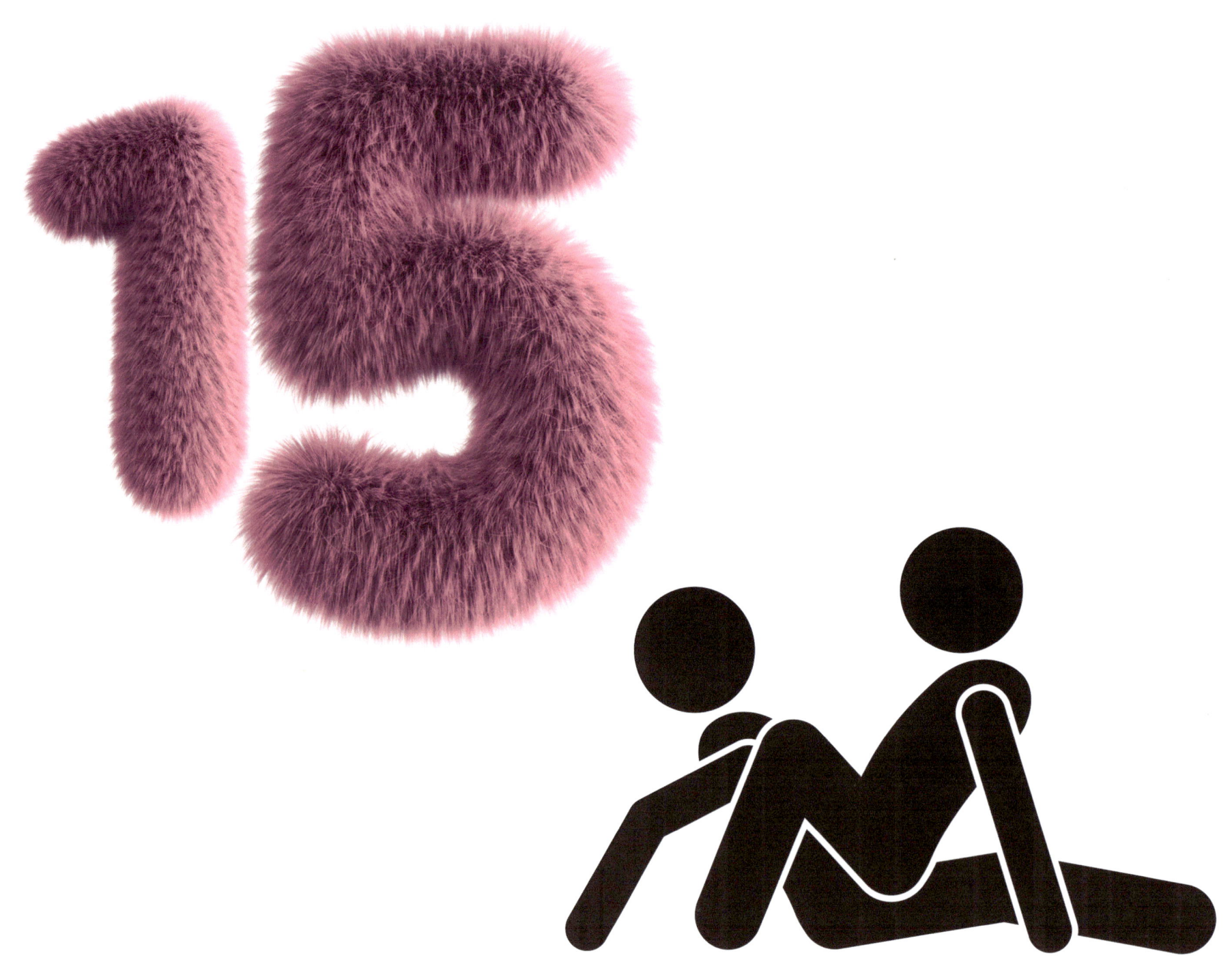

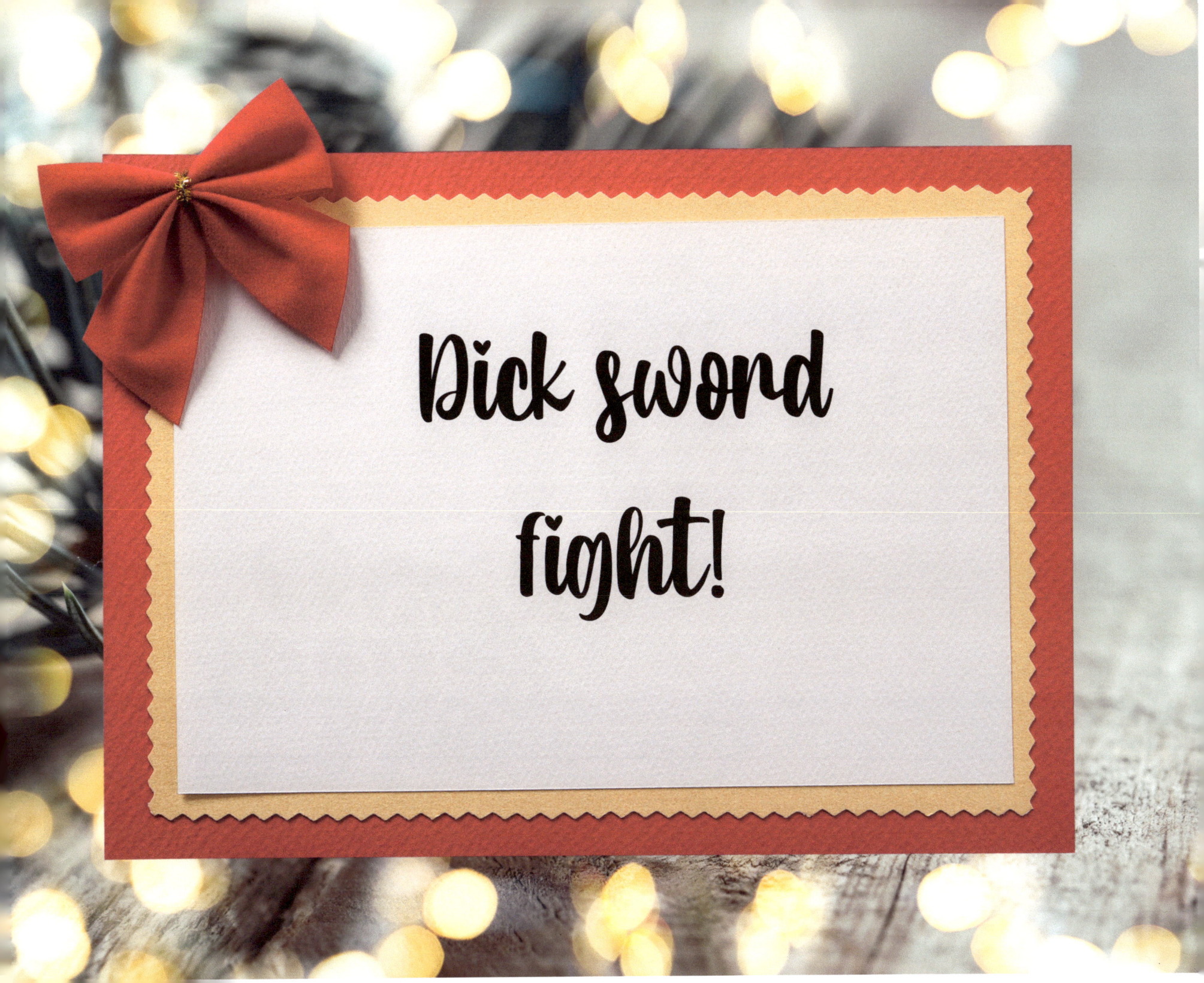

16

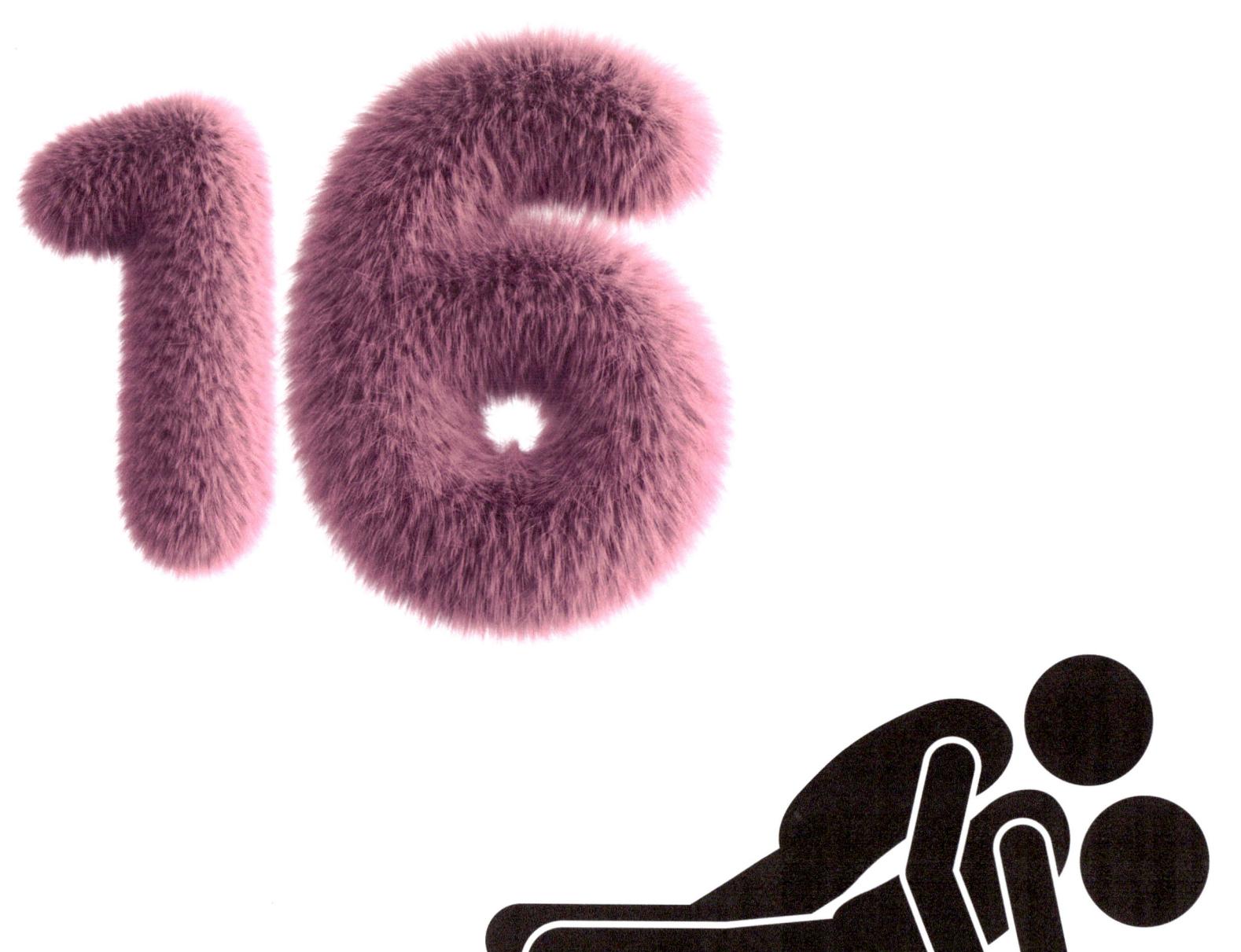

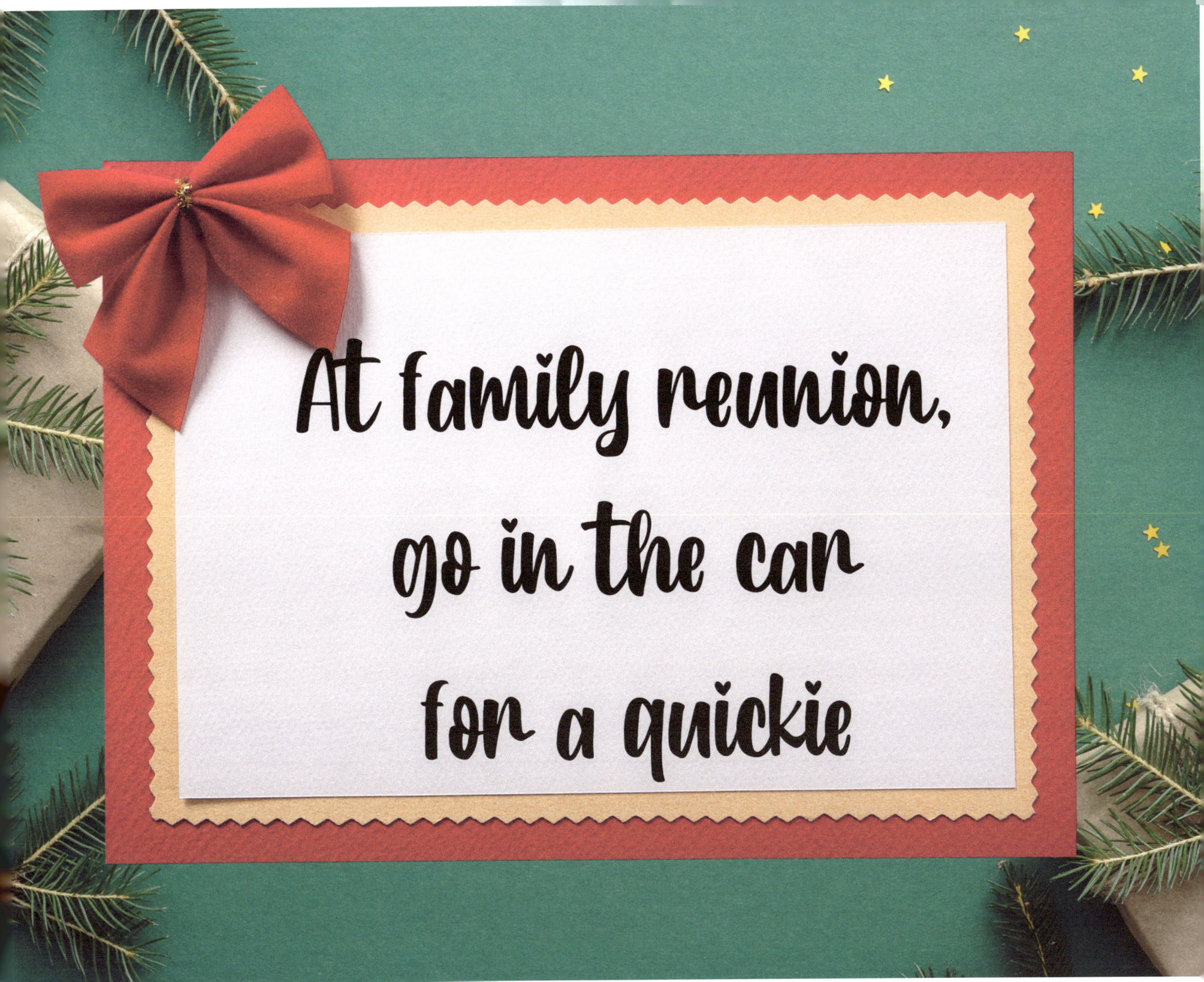

17

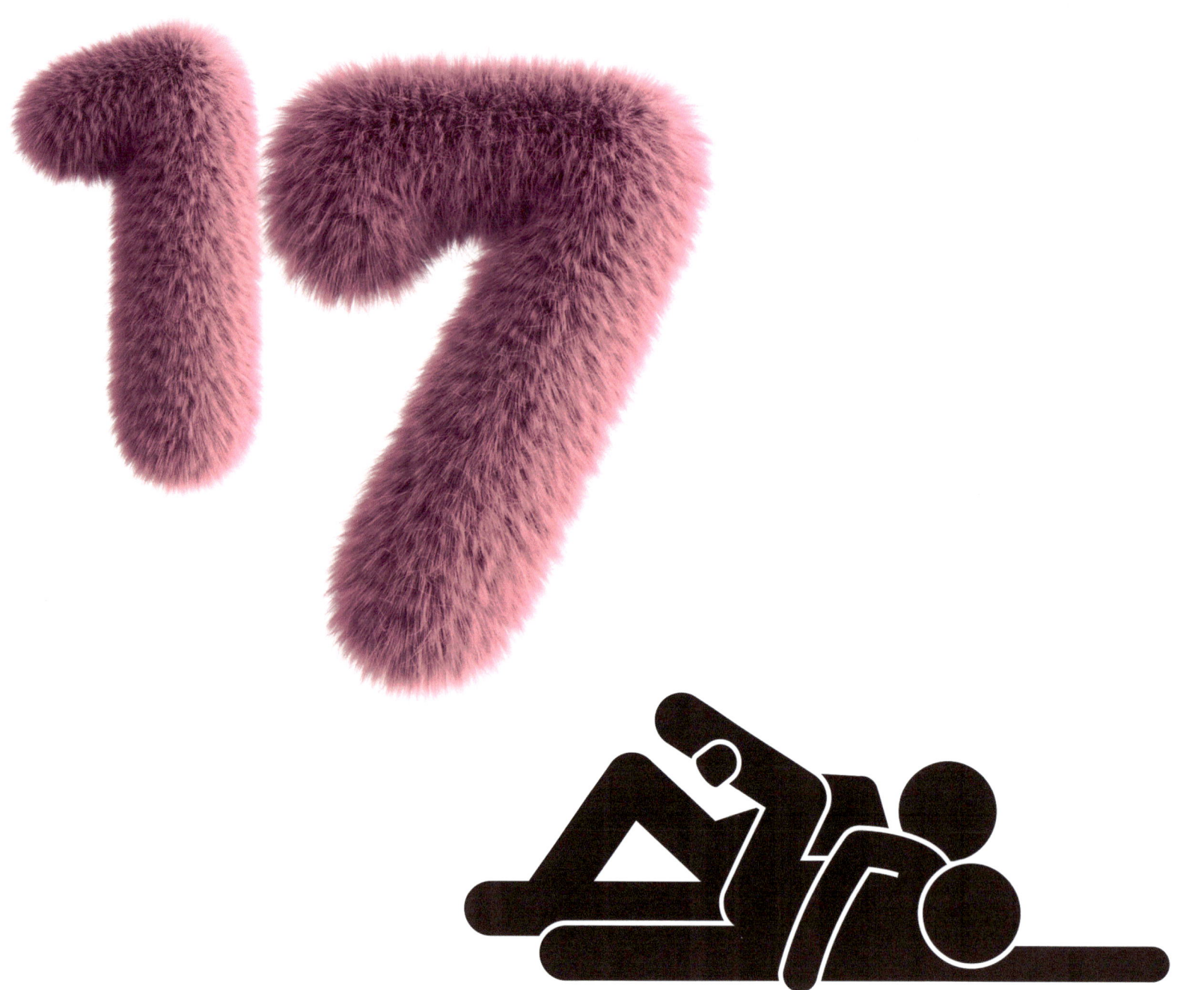

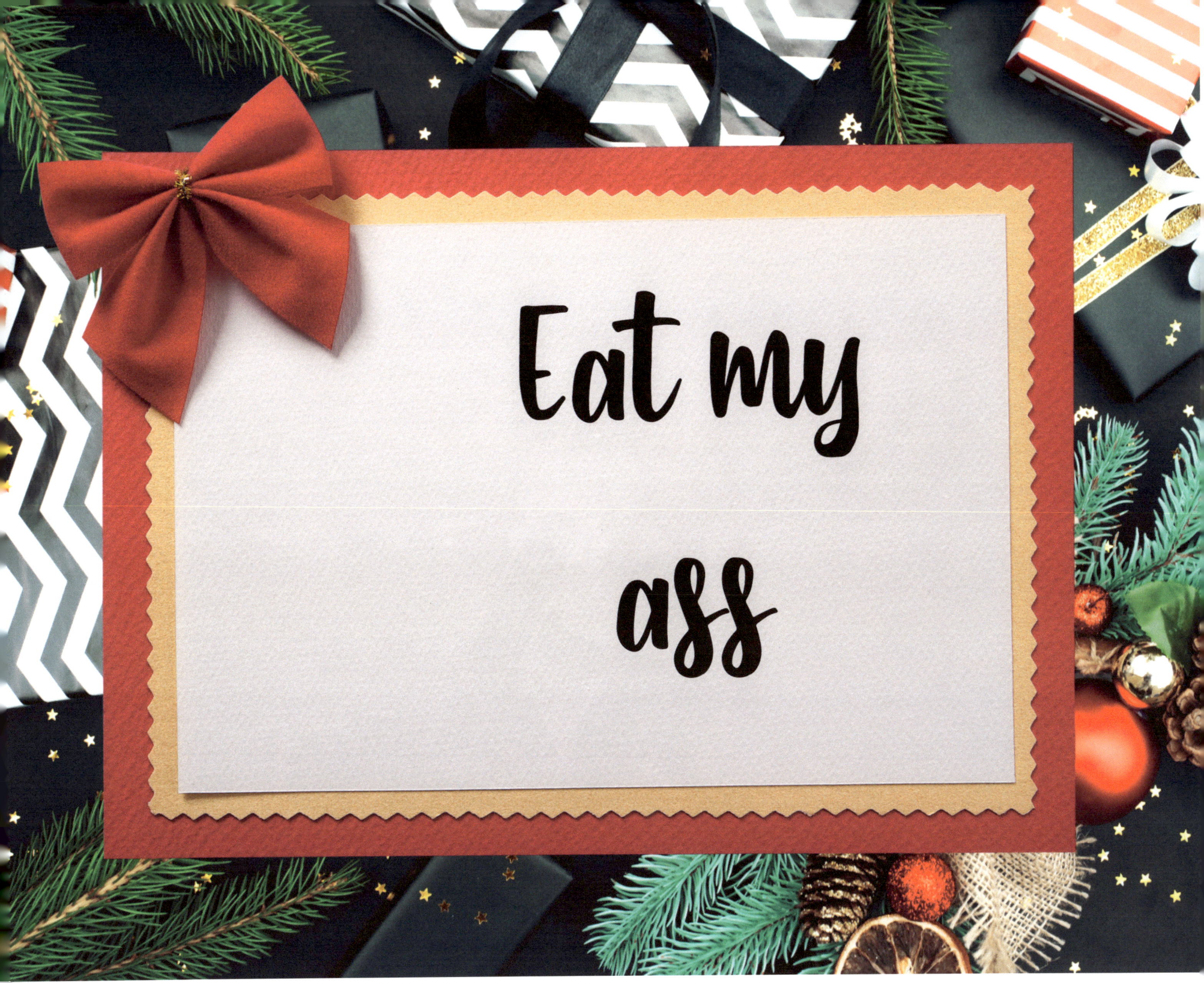

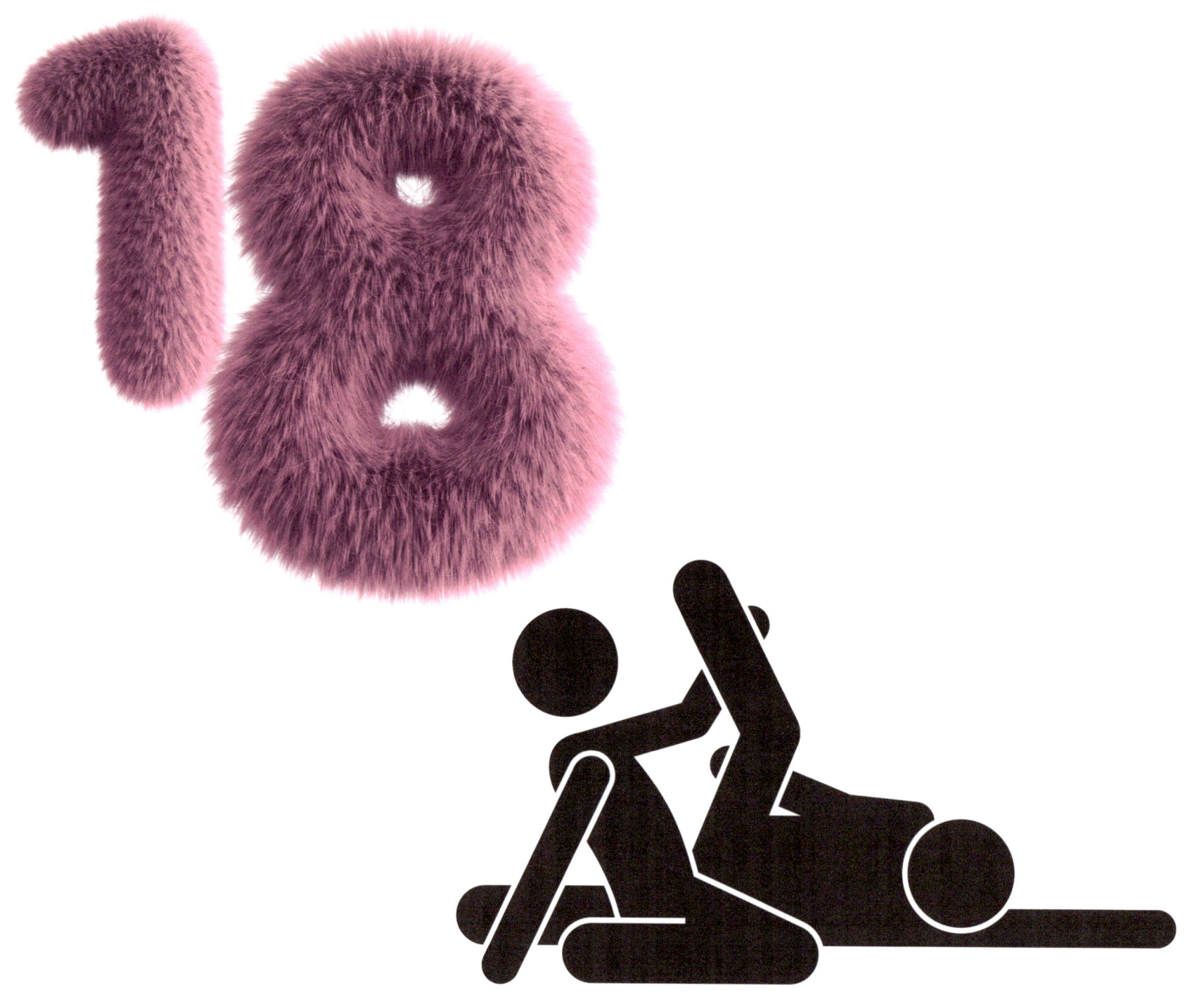

Sex at the cinema

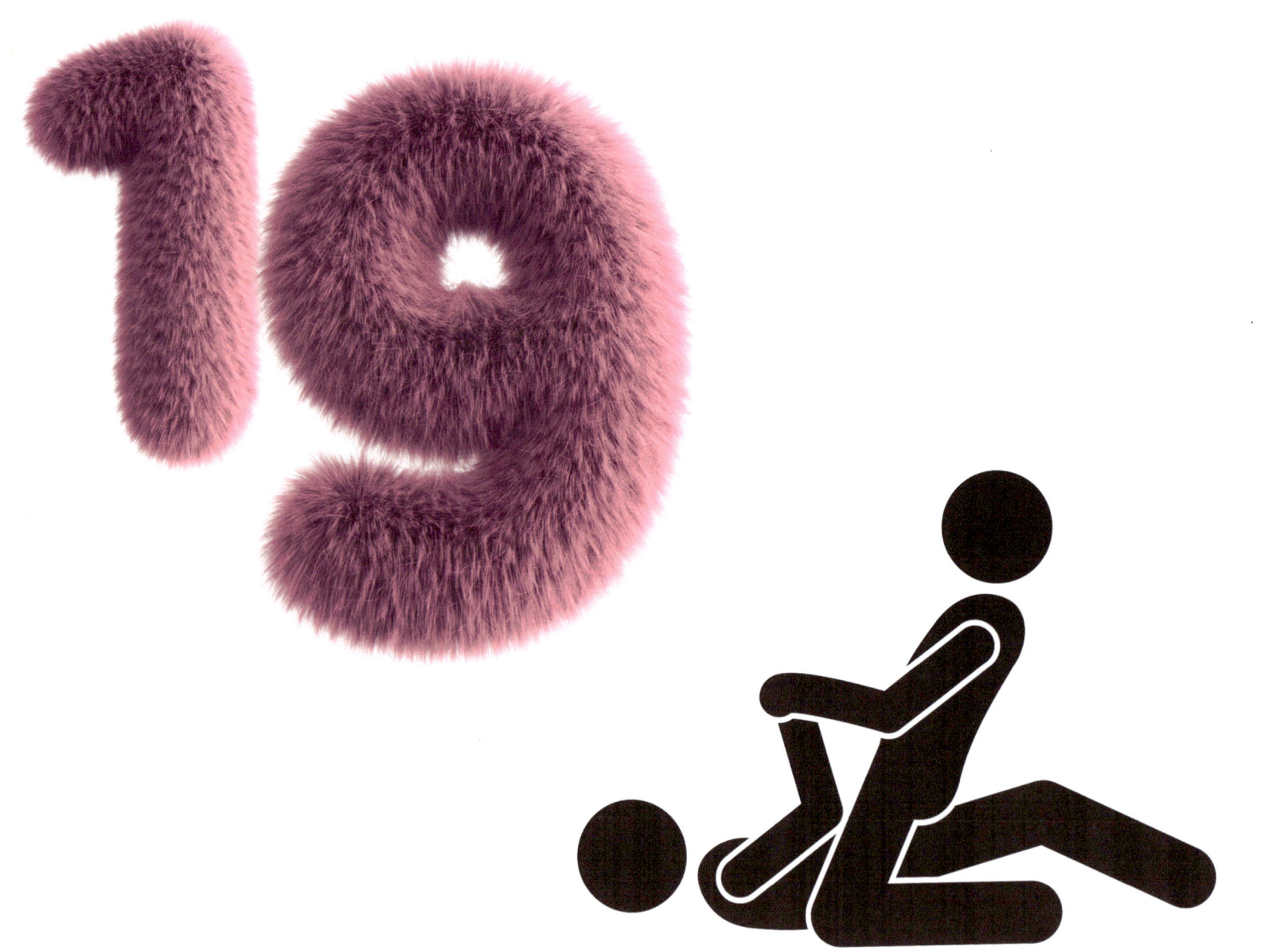

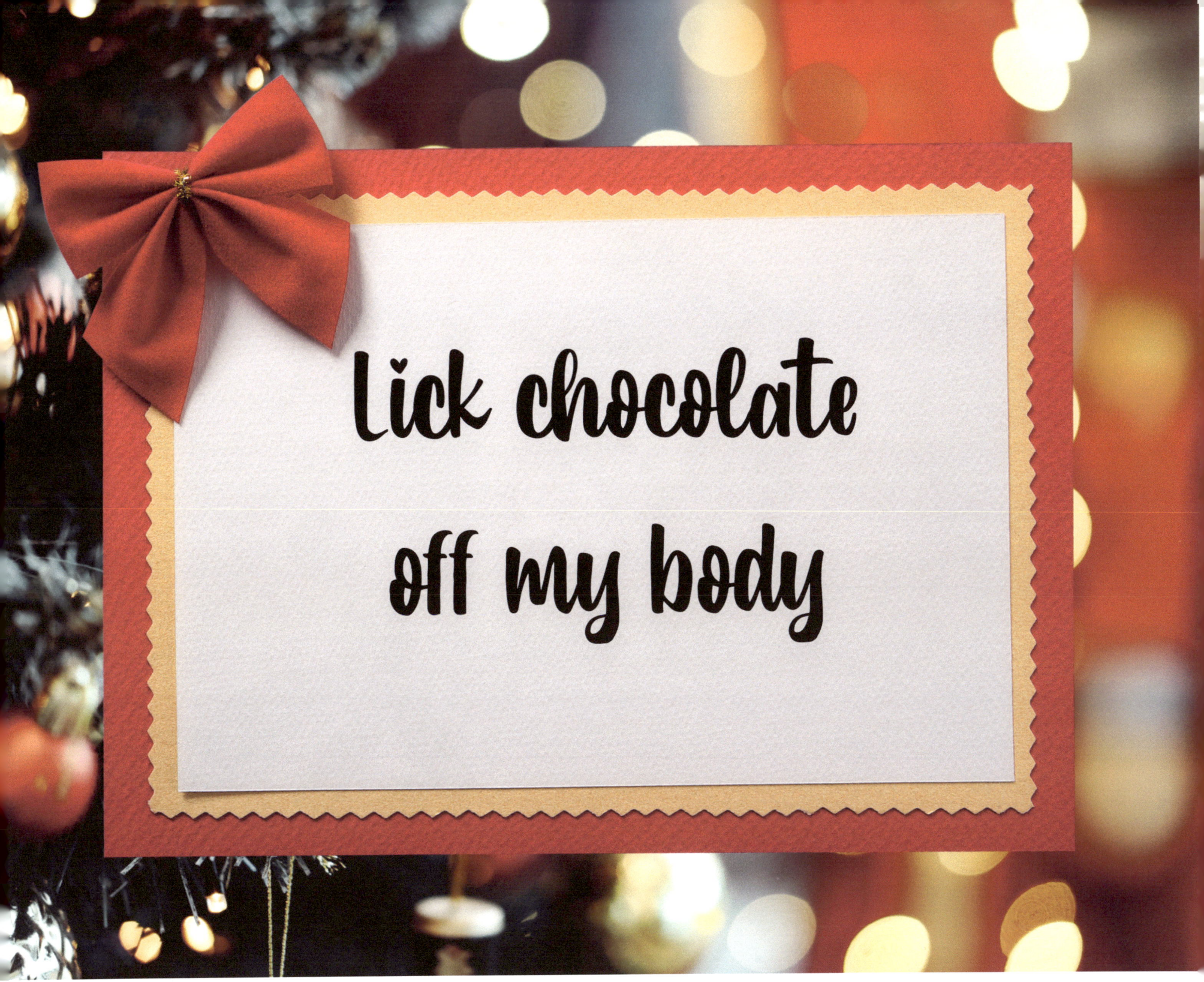

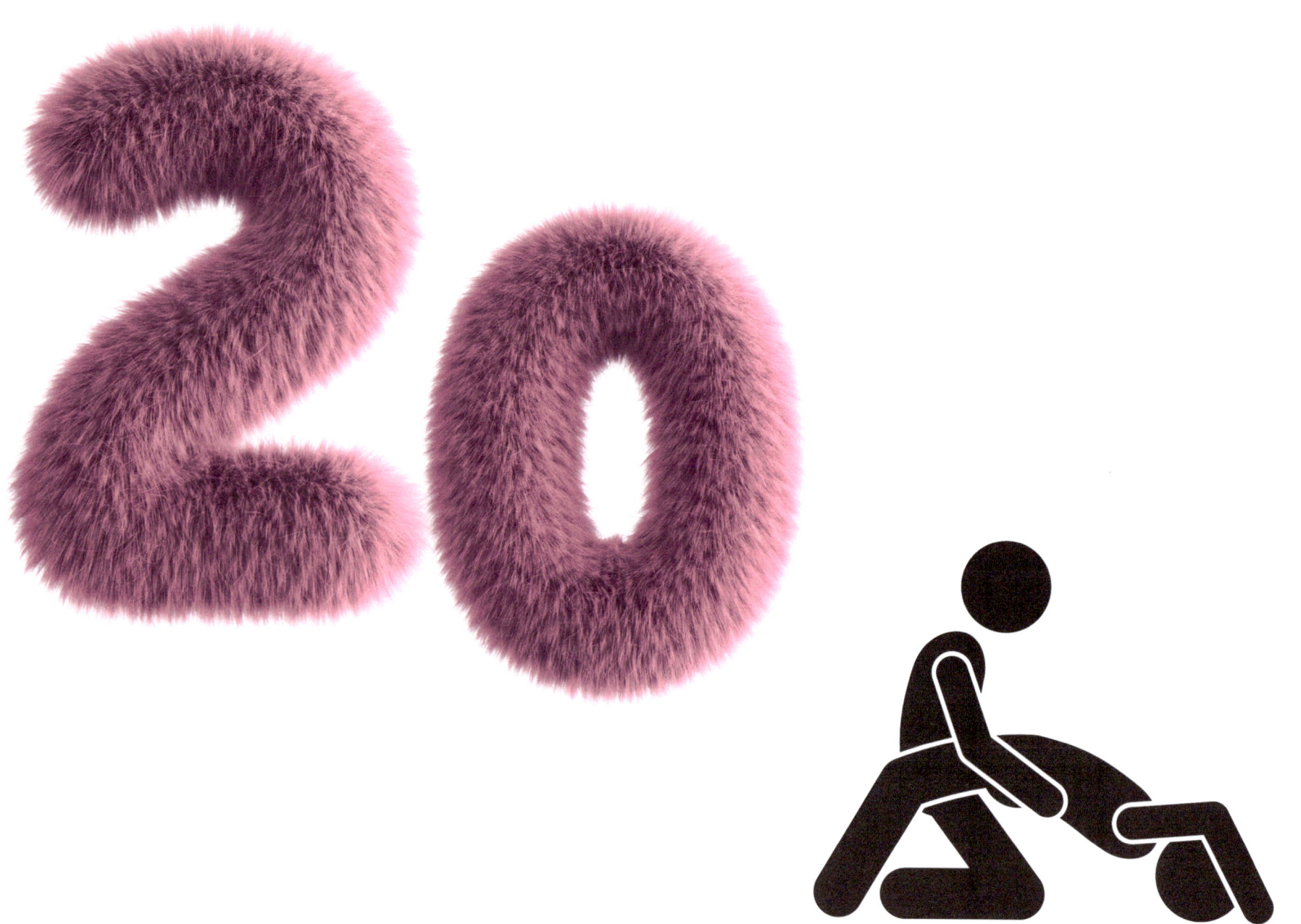

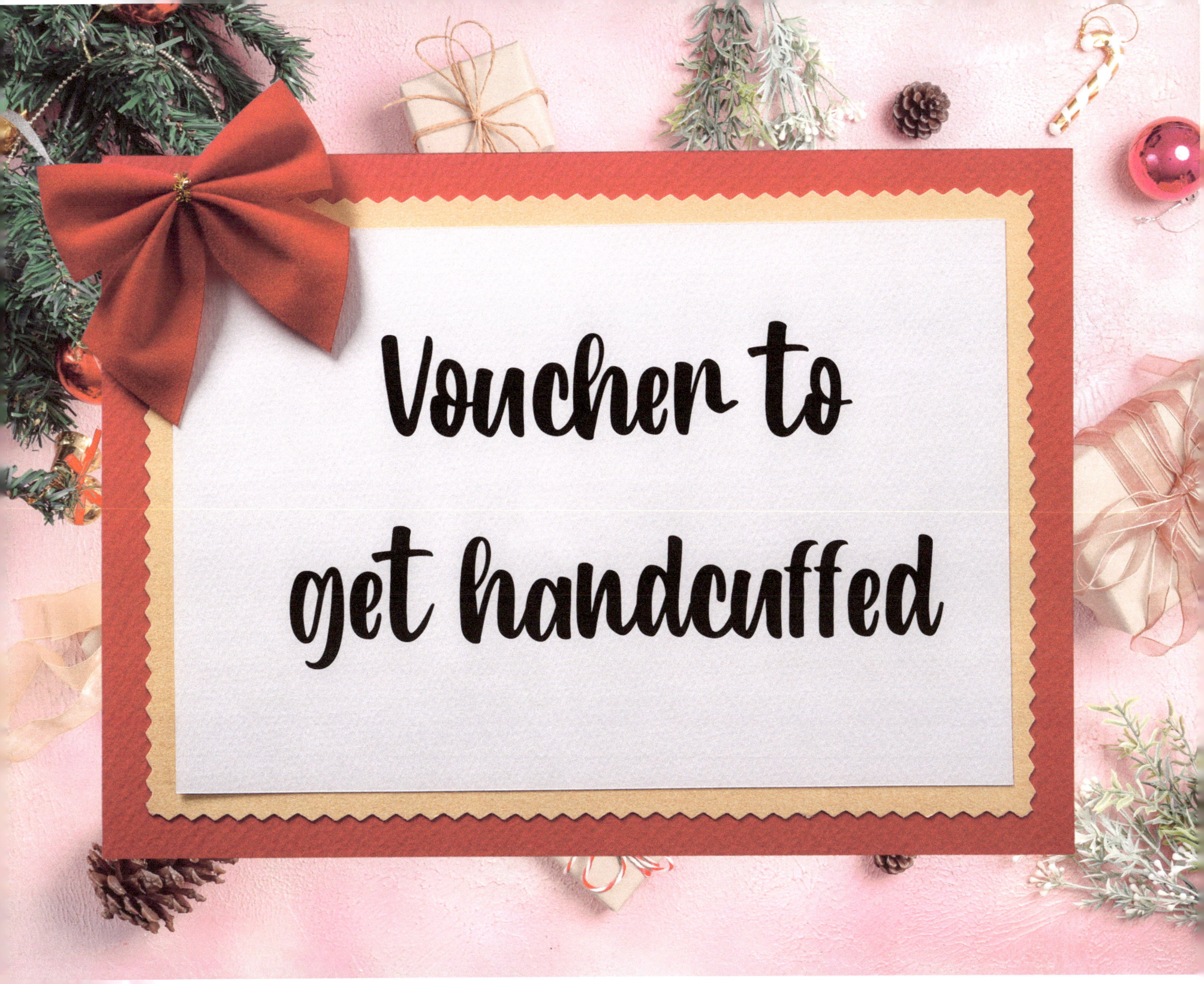

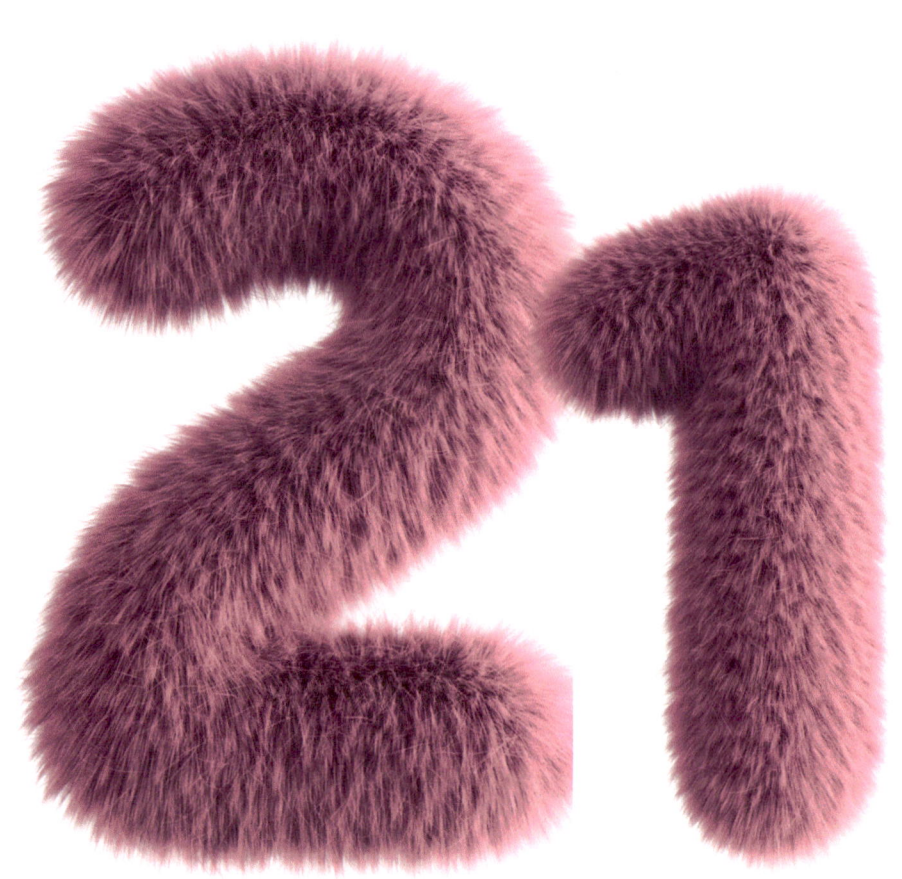

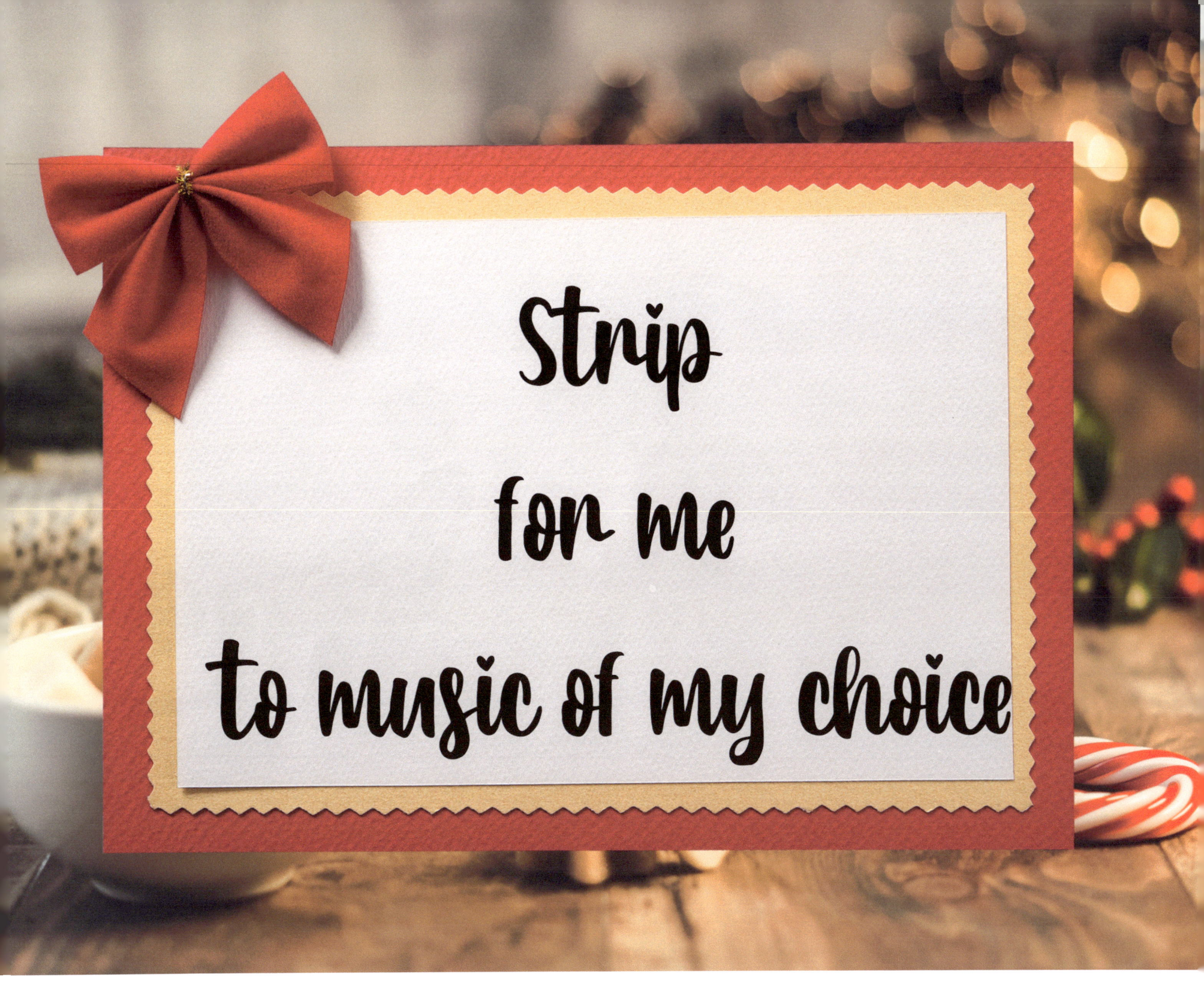

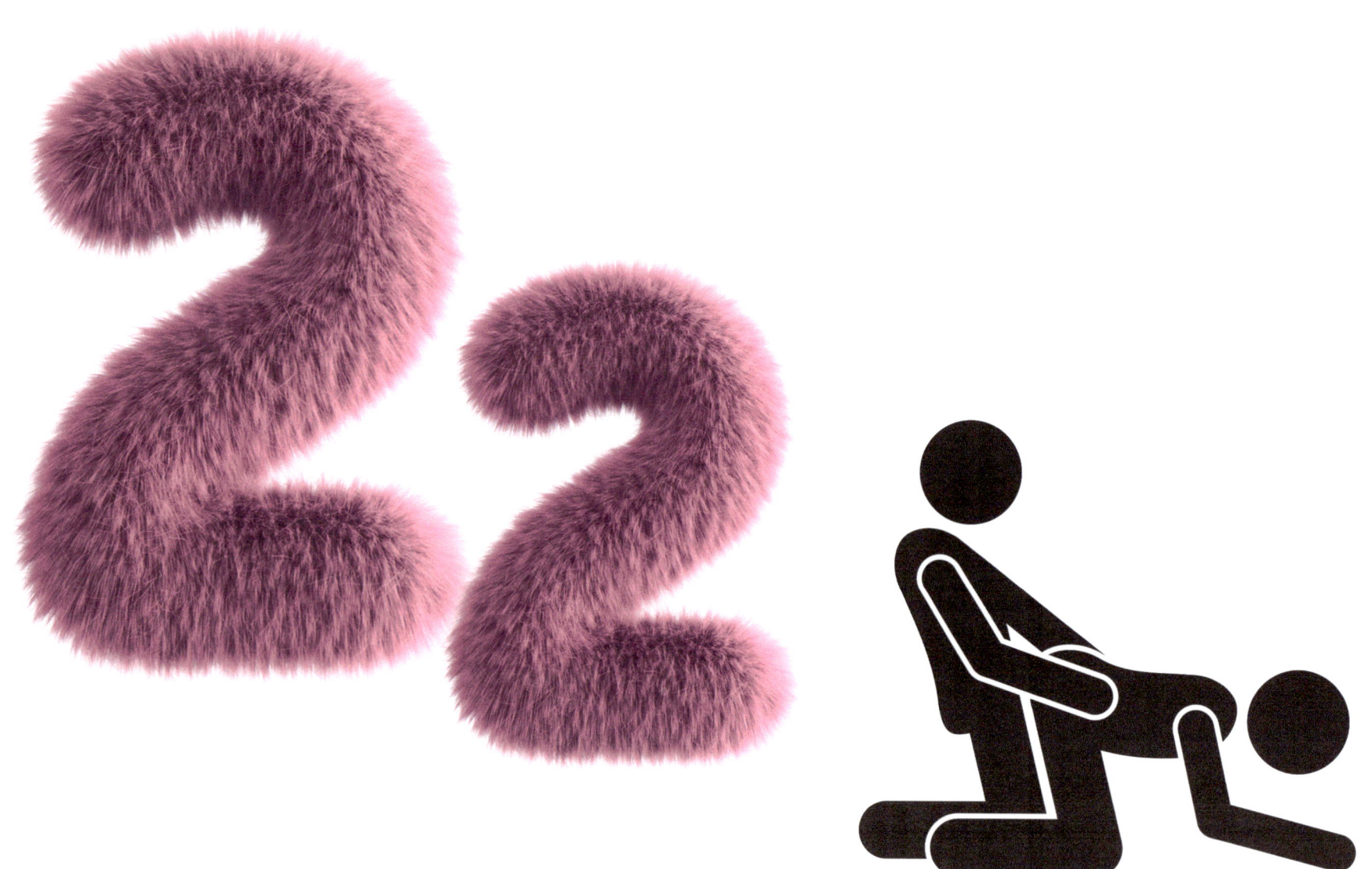

Sex with without curtains being drawn

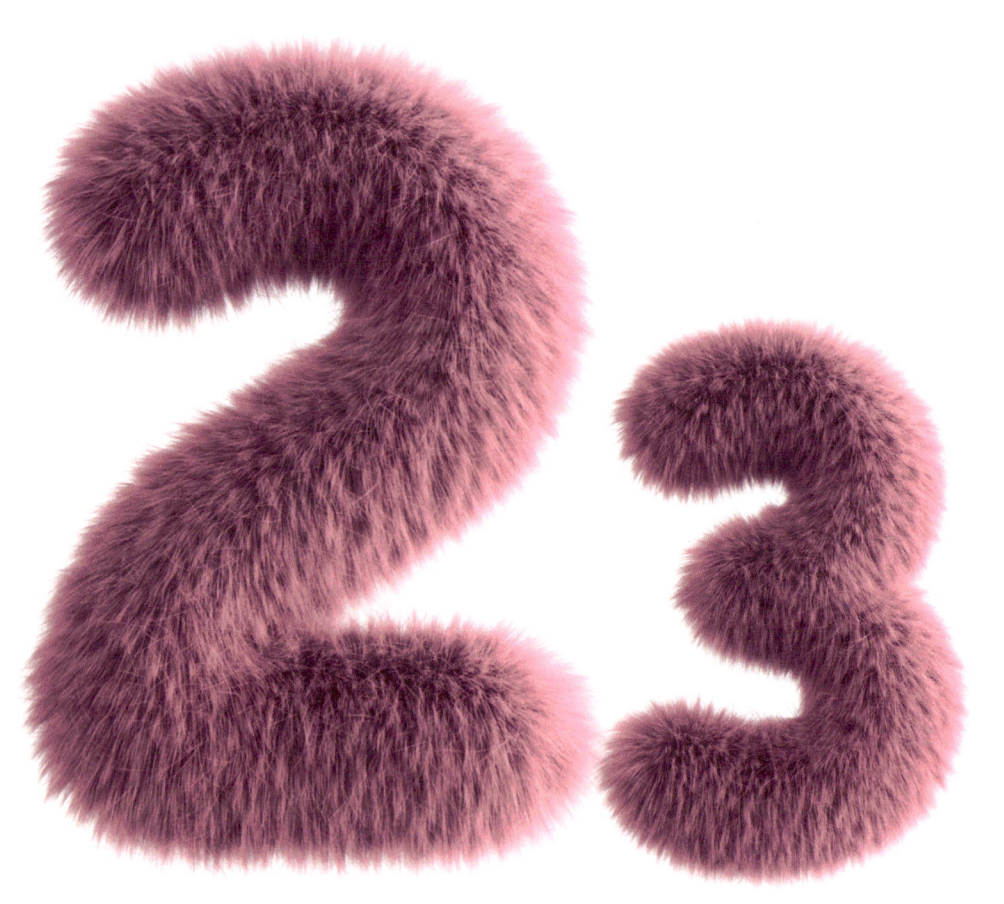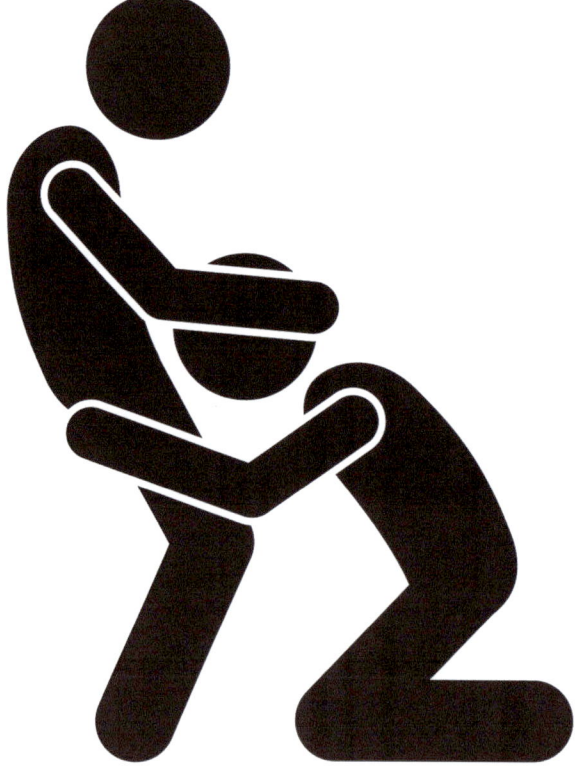

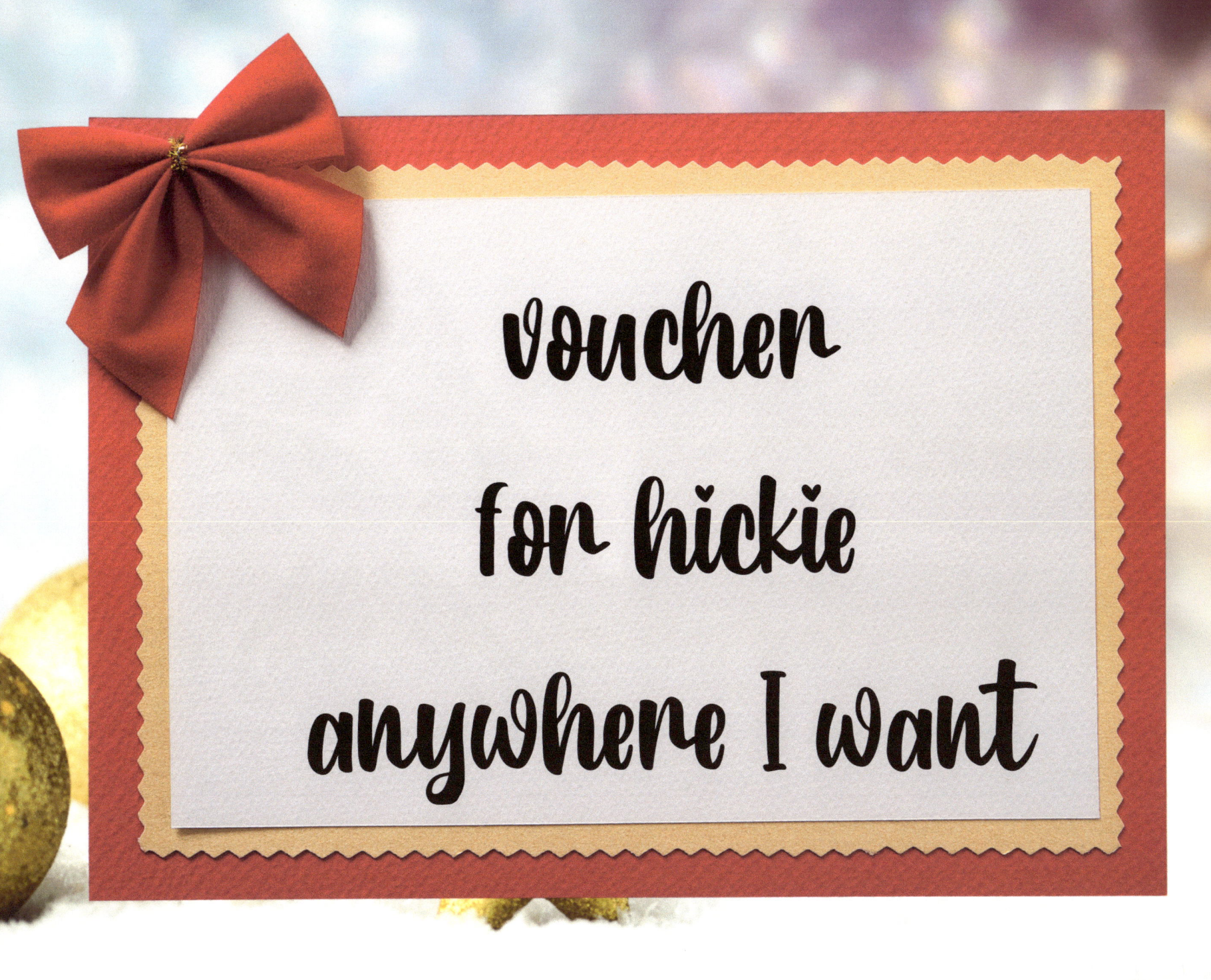

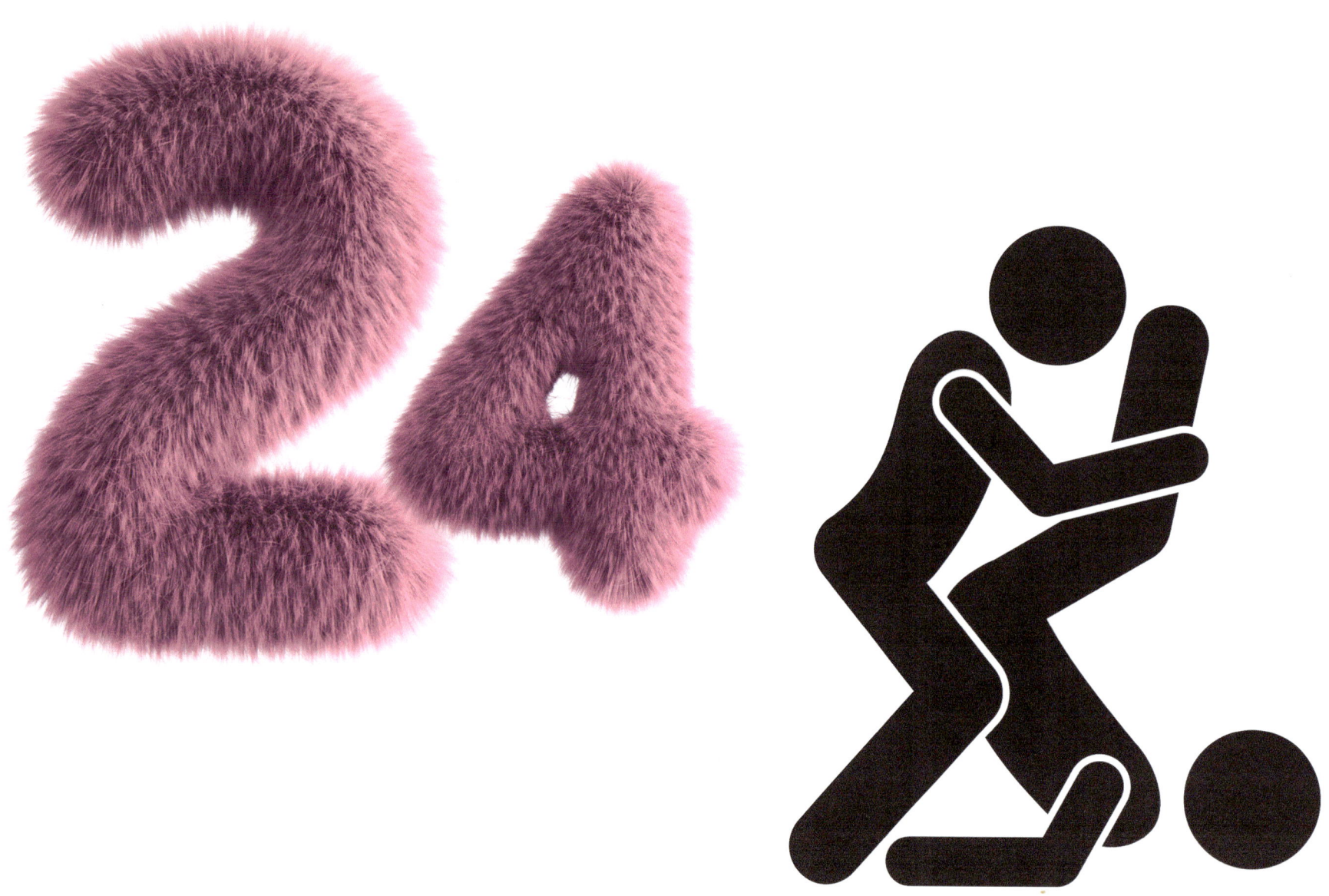

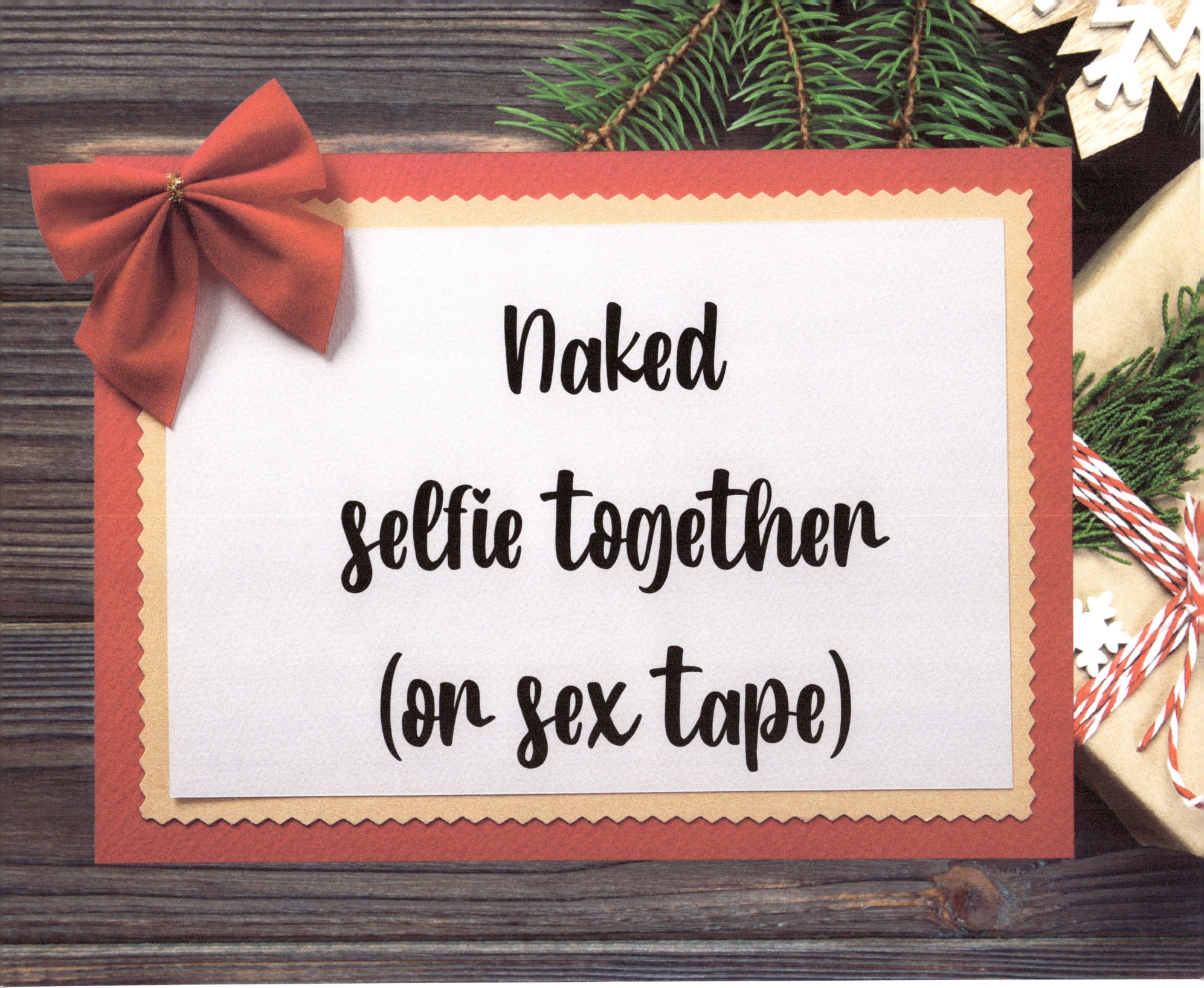

25

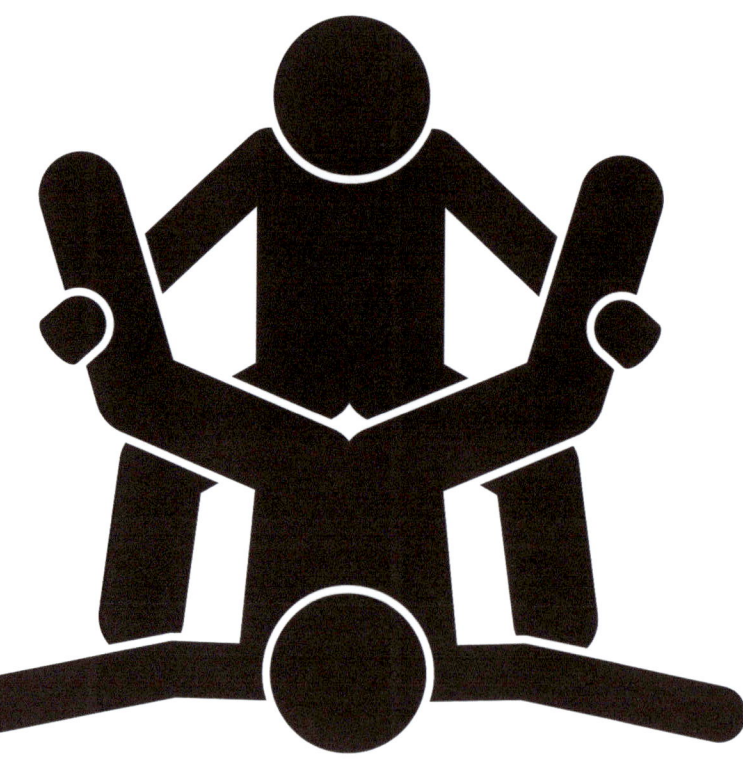

www.ingramcontent.com/pod-product-compliance
Lightning Source LLC
Chambersburg PA
CBHW042035120526

44592CB00028B/64